SPIRITUAL YOGA

BOOKS by
His Divine Grace A. C. Bhaktivedanta Swami Prabhupāda

Bhagavad-gītā As It Is
Śrīmad-Bhāgavatam (completed by disciples)
Śrī Caitanya-caritāmṛta
Kṛṣṇa, the Supreme Personality of Godhead
Teachings of Lord Caitanya
The Nectar of Devotion
The Nectar of Instruction
Śrī Īśopaniṣad
Light of the Bhāgavata
Easy Journey to Other Planets
Teachings of Lord Kapila, the Son of Devahūti
Teachings of Queen Kuntī
Message of Godhead
The Science of Self-Realization
The Perfection of Yoga
Beyond Birth and Death
On the Way to Kṛṣṇa
Rāja-vidyā: The King of Knowledge
Elevation to Kṛṣṇa Consciousness
Kṛṣṇa Consciousness: The Matchless Gift
Kṛṣṇa Consciousness: The Topmost Yoga System
Perfect Questions, Perfect Answers
Life Comes from Life
The Nārada-bhakti-sūtra (completed by disciples)
The Mukunda-mālā-stotra (completed by disciples)
Geetār-gān (Bengali)
Vairāgya-vidyā (Bengali)
Buddhi-yoga (Bengali)
Bhakti-ratna-boli (Bengali)
Back to Godhead magazine (founder)

BOOKS compiled from the teachings of His Divine Grace
A. C. Bhaktivedanta Swami Prabhupāda after his lifetime

Search for Liberation
A Second Chance
The Journey of Self-Discovery
Civilization and Transcendence
The Laws of Nature
Renunciation Through Wisdom
The Quest for Enlightenment
Dharma, the Way of Transcendence
Beyond Illusion and Doubt
The Hare Kṛṣṇa Challenge
Spiritual Yoga
Bhakti, the Art of Eternal Love

THE PATH TO THE HIGHEST PLEASURE

SPIRITUAL YOGA

HIS DIVINE GRACE
A. C. Bhaktivedanta Swami Prabhupāda
Founder-Ācārya of the International Society for Krishna Consciousness

THE BHAKTIVEDANTA BOOK TRUST
Los Angeles • London • Stockholm • Mumbai • Sydney • Hong Kong

Readers interested in the subject matter of this book are invited by the International Society for Krishna Consciousness to correspond with its secretary.

International Society for Krishna Consciousness
P.O. Box 34074
Los Angeles, California 90034, USA
Telephone: 1-800-927-4152 (Inside USA); 1-310-837-5283 (Outside USA)
Fax: 1-310-837-1056
e-mail: bbt.usa@krishna.com
web: www.krishna.com

International Society for Krishna Consciousness
P.O. Box 380
Riverstone, NSW 2765, Australia
Telephone: +61-2-9627-6306
Fax: +61-2-9627-6052
e-mail: bbt.au@krishna.com

Design: Arcita Dāsa
Cover Painting: "Lord Ṛṣabhadeva Instructs His sons," by Locana Dāsa

First Printing, 2004: 100,000

Printed in Australia

ISBN 0-89213-330-9

CONTENTS

INTRODUCTION

There's one kind of yoga for the body, and there's another kind of yoga for the soul. This book is about the yoga for the soul. It's called *bhakti-yoga,* the yoga of pure love and devotion, the yoga of the highest pleasure.

The yoga of the body is the kind most people know about, the kind that is on the covers of the magazines. Everybody knows about that. But the yoga of the soul is something new for most people. You can only find it deep inside of you.

In the yoga of the body, you can stretch your body muscles, and feel good for some time. With the yoga of the soul, you stretch your soul muscles, and feel good forever. That's the difference. And that is what this book is all about.

Now there's nothing wrong with the yoga of the body, but when you are ready for the ultimate yoga, the spiritual yoga of the soul is waiting for you. And it's been waiting for a long time. Way before the first teacher of body yoga came to the yoga studios of the West, the teachers of spiritual yoga were sitting in mountains and forests of ancient India teaching their favored students their secrets for attaining the highest pleasure.

For those who really know, that is the highest goal. But to get to it, you have to know the path. And you can find that out only from the knower of the path, the teacher of spiritual yoga.

One of these teachers was Śrī Ṛṣabhadeva. *Deva* means "God." Although He appeared like an ordinary human, He was a form of God and so had divine powers. He lived long ago—millions of years ago, in fact. Externally, He appeared like a great king, which means He had every chance to enjoy to the hilt every kind of material pleasure. But just to set the perfect example of self-control, He did not. He taught the techniques of spiritual yoga to His sons, and then this secret knowledge, the path to the highest pleasure, was passed down through the generations from one spiritual master to another.

For many ages, this secret knowledge was never written down. It was kept hidden in memory, and revealed only to the proper candidates. As time passed, people's power of memory began to decline. Therefore, about five thousand years ago, a great spiritual personality named Vyāsadeva put the teachings of Ṛṣabha in writing, as part of a Sanskrit book called *Śrīmad-Bhāgavatam*. Still, for a long time afterwards only a chosen few in India learned about these teachings.

Then in the late twentieth century, His Divine Grace A. C. Bhaktivedanta Swami Prabhupāda, the greatest spiritual master of the modern age, following the orders of his own spiritual master, translated Ṛṣabha's teachings on spiritual yoga into English and brought them to the Western world, giving you the chance to enter onto the path to the highest pleasure.

This book is a combination of Śrīla Prabhupāda's published translation and commentary on the original Sanskrit teachings of Ṛṣabha (*Śrīmad-Bhāgavatam* 5.5.1–14) and the transcripts of a series of lectures he gave on these teachings in various cities (including London, Stockholm, and Vṛndāvana, India) during the years 1969 to 1976.

We hope you enjoy the teachings of Ṛṣabhadeva on spiritual yoga, the path to the highest pleasure.

The Editors

1: Don't Be Like Hogs and Dogs

ṛṣabha uvāca
nāyaṁ deho deha-bhājāṁ nṛloke
kaṣṭān kāmān arhate viḍ-bhujāṁ ye
tapo divyaṁ putrakā yena sattvaṁ
śuddhyed yasmād brahma-saukhyaṁ tv anantam

Lord Ṛṣabhadeva told His sons: My dear boys, of all the living entities who have accepted material bodies in this world, one who has been awarded this human form should not work hard day and night simply for sense gratification, which is available even for dogs and for hogs that eat stool. One should engage in penance and austerity to attain the divine position of devotional service. By such activity, one's heart is purified, and when one attains this position, he attains eternal, blissful life, which is transcendental to material happiness and which continues forever.

Śrīmad-Bhāgavatam 5.5.1

In this verse Lord Ṛṣabhadeva tells His sons about the importance of human life. The word *deha-bhāk* refers to anyone who accepts a material body, but the living entity who is awarded the human form must act differently from animals. Animals like dogs and hogs enjoy sense gratification by eating stool. After undergoing severe hardships all day, human beings are trying to enjoy themselves at night by eating, drinking, having sex, and sleeping. At the same time, they have to properly defend themselves. However, this is not human civilization. Human life means voluntarily practicing suffering for the advancement of spiritual life. There is, of course, suffering in the lives of animals and plants, which are suffering due to their past misdeeds. However, human beings should voluntarily accept suffering in the form of austerities and penances in order to attain the divine life. After attaining the divine life, one can enjoy happiness eternally. After all, every living entity is trying to enjoy happiness, but as long as one is encaged in the material body, he has to suffer different kinds of misery. A higher sense is present in the human form. We should act according to superior advice in order to attain eternal happiness and go back to Godhead.

It is significant in this verse that the government and the natural guardian, the father, should educate subordinates and raise them to Kṛṣṇa consciousness. When devoid of Kṛṣṇa consciousness, living beings suffer in the cycle of birth and death perpetually. To relieve them from this bondage and enable them to become blissful and happy, *bhakti-yoga,* or Kṛṣṇa consciousness, should be taught. A foolish civilization neglects to teach people how to rise to the platform of *bhakti-yoga.* Without Kṛṣṇa consciousness a person is no better than a hog or dog. The instructions of Ṛṣabhadeva are very essential at the present moment. People are being educated and trained to work very hard for sense gratification, and there is no sublime aim in life. A man travels to earn his livelihood, leaving home early in the morning, catching a local train and being packed in a compartment. He has to stand for an hour or two in order to reach his place of business. Then again he takes a bus to get to the office. At the office he works hard from nine to five; then he takes two or three hours to return home. After eating, he has sex and goes to sleep. For all this hardship, his only happiness is a little sex. *Yan maithunādi-gṛhamedhi-sukhaṁ hi tuccham.* Ṛṣabhadeva clearly states that human life is not meant for this kind of existence, which is enjoyed even by dogs and hogs. Indeed, dogs and hogs do not have to work so hard for sex. A human being should try to live in a different way and should not try to imitate dogs and hogs. The alternative is mentioned. Human life is meant for *tapasya*—austerity and penance. By *tapasya,* one can get out of the material clutches. When one is situated in Kṛṣṇa consciousness, devotional service, his happiness is guaranteed eternally. By taking to *bhakti-yoga,* devotional service, one's existence is purified. The living entity is seeking happiness life after life, but he can make a solution to all his problems simply by practicing *bhakti-yoga.* Then he immediately becomes eligible to return home, back to Godhead. As Lord Kṛṣṇa confirms in the *Bhagavad-gītā* (4.9):

janma karma ca me divyam evaṁ yo vetti tattvataḥ
tyaktvā dehaṁ punar janma naiti mām eti so 'rjuna

"One who knows the transcendental nature of My appearance and activities does not, upon leaving the body, take his birth again in this material world, but attains My eternal abode, O Arjuna."

Now the question might be "What is the meaning of *tapasya*—austerities and penances?" *Tapasya* means voluntarily agreeing to mold your life according to the rules and regulations given by the scriptures, the spiritual master, and saintly persons. So Lord Ṛṣabhadeva is instructing His sons, "My dear sons, don't spoil your life by living like cats and dogs and hogs. Utilize your valuable human life by accepting *tapasya.*"

The question may then be "Why this injunction? Why should I not live like an animal? Why do I have to live under the regulative principles of scriptures and saintly persons and the spiritual master?" Ṛṣabhadeva answers, *tapo divyaṁ putrakā yena sattvaṁ śuddhyet:* "My dear sons, if you accept this principle of *tapasya,* your existence will be purified." At present we are contaminated by the modes of material nature, mostly ignorance and passion. So Ṛṣabhadeva is advising his sons that if they abide by the instructions of scripture and so on, they will be purified of the lower modes of nature.

Then the question may be "What is the use of purifying one's existence?" Ṛṣabhadeva answers, *yasmād brahma-saukhyaṁ tv anantam.* "When your existence is purified, you will be situated on the transcendental platform of blissful life, which is eternal." You are hankering after happiness. Why are you struggling so hard in this material existence? For happiness. Why are you after sense gratification? For happiness. Why do you want to possess so many things? For happiness. Why do you want to become beautiful? For happiness. Why do you want to eat so many things? For happiness. In every endeavor, happiness is your ultimate goal. But the happiness you are now deriving from material sources is temporary. You may become happy by intoxication, but for how long? That happiness is temporary. You may become happy by sex indulgence, but for how long? That happiness lasts for a few minutes or a few seconds. So if you want eternal, continuous happiness, you have to purify your existential condition and place yourself in the transcendental position; then you will enjoy eternal happiness.

This happiness is described in the *Padma Purāṇa* as follows:

ramante yogino 'nante satyānande cid-ātmani
iti rāma-padenāsau paraṁ brahmābhidhīyate

"The Supreme Absolute Truth is called Rāma because the transcendentalists enjoy [*ramante*] the unlimited true happiness of spiritual existence." So the transcendentalists are also enjoying sense gratification. But how? By serving the sense gratification of the Supreme, Param Brahma. *Ramante* means "to enjoy sense gratification." For example, one of Kṛṣṇa's names is Rādhā-ramaṇa, "He who enjoys sense gratification with His eternal consort, Rādhārāṇī." So sense gratification is there in the transcendental position, but not this material sense gratification. Material sense gratification is a perverted reflection of spiritual sense gratification.

Devotional service is spiritual sense gratification: *hṛṣīkeṇa hṛṣīkeśa-sevanam*. *Hṛṣīka* means "senses," and Hṛṣīkeśa means "the master of the senses." The master of the senses is Kṛṣṇa. So when you use your senses for Kṛṣṇa's sense gratification, you are in the transcendental position. And when you use your senses for your own sense gratification, that is material. This is the difference. So when you are situated on the transcendental platform, when your existence is purified by *tapasya*—by voluntarily accepting austerity and penance under the guidance of the spiritual master, the scriptures, and saintly persons—at that time you will become fully satisfied by satisfying the senses of Kṛṣṇa.

The process is something like how the various parts of the body are nourished when we eat food. The different parts of the body depend on the stomach to enjoy food; they cannot enjoy food independently. Suppose you pick up a nice piece of cake with your fingers—the fingers cannot enjoy it independently. But if the fingers put it into the mouth and it goes to the stomach, then the stomach digests it and it turns into blood, and the heart circulates the blood to the different parts of the body, and your fingers are nourished. This is the process by which the fingers can enjoy the cake. Similarly, in devotional service sense gratification is there—but through serving Kṛṣṇa. Then you will feel complete satisfaction.

So real human life means to purify our present existential condition by voluntarily accepting the regulative principles given by the spiritual master, the scriptures, and the saintly persons. And when we become purified by employing our senses in the service of the Supreme Lord, we actually enjoy our senses.

2: Serve the Great Souls

mahat-sevāṁ dvāram āhur vimuktes
tamo-dvāraṁ yoṣitāṁ saṅgi-saṅgam
mahāntas te sama-cittāḥ praśāntā
vimanyavaḥ suhṛdaḥ sādhavo ye

One can attain the path of liberation from material bondage only by rendering service to highly advanced spiritual personalities. These personalities are impersonalists and devotees. Whether one wants to merge into the Lord's existence or wants to associate with the Personality of Godhead, one should render service to the mahātmās. For those who are not interested in such activities, who associate with people fond of women and sex, the path to hell is wide open. The mahātmās are equipoised. They do not see any difference between one living entity and another. They are very peaceful and are fully engaged in devotional service. They are devoid of anger, and they work for the benefit of everyone. They do not behave in any abominable way. Such people are known as mahātmās.

Śrīmad-Bhāgavatam 5.5.2

The human body is like a junction. One may take either the path of liberation or the path leading to a hellish condition. How one can take these paths is described herein. On the path of liberation one associates with *mahātmās,* and on the path of bondage one associates with those attached to sense gratification and women. There are two types of *mahātmās*—the impersonalist and the devotee. Although their ultimate goal is different, the process of emancipation is almost the same. Both want eternal happiness. One seeks happiness in impersonal Brahman, and the other seeks happiness in the association of the Supreme Personality of Godhead. This happiness is described in the first verse as *brahma-saukhyam.* Brahman means "spirit" or "the eternal"; both the impersonalist and the devotee seek eternal blissful life. In any case, it is advised that one become perfect. In the words of *Caitanya-caritāmṛta* (*Madhya* 22.87):

asat-saṅga-tyāga,—ei vaiṣṇava-ācāra
'strī-saṅgī'—eka asādhu, 'kṛṣṇābhakta' āra

To remain unattached to the modes of material nature, one should avoid associating with those who are *asat,* materialistic. There are two kinds of materialists. One is attached to women and sense gratification, and the other is simply a nondevotee. On the positive side is association with *mahātmās,* and on the negative side is the avoidance of nondevotees and woman-hunters.

Who is a *mahātmā,* a great soul? In the *Bhagavad-gītā* (9.13) Kṛṣṇa says, *mahātmānas tu māṁ pārtha daivīṁ prakṛtim āśritāḥ.* A great soul is one who has taken shelter of God's spiritual nature, or spiritual energy. God has two energies, the material energy and the spiritual energy, and from the presence of these energies we can understand that God exists, just as we can understand from the presence of the sunlight that the sun has risen in the sky. Light is simply the energy of the sun, so in the morning, as soon as you look through your window and see that there is light in the sky, you can understand that the sun has risen. Similarly, we can understand the existence of God by the presence of His spiritual and material energies. Otherwise, where have these energies come from? As stated in the *Viṣṇu Purāṇa:*

ekadeśa-sthitasyāgner jyotsnā vistāriṇī yathā
parasya brahmaṇaḥ śaktis tathedam akhilaṁ jagat

"Just as a fire situated in one place spreads its illumination all over, so the Supreme Personality of Godhead, Parabrahman, spreads His energies all over this universe." So in this verse spoken by Ṛṣabhadeva the words *mahat* and *mahāntas* refer to the *mahātmās,* those who have taken shelter of the Lord's spiritual energy. If one wants to be liberated from the entanglement of material life—from the miseries of birth, death, old age, and disease and so many other sufferings—one has to serve such a great saintly person and execute austerities under his direction.

And how can you understand who has taken shelter of the Lord's spiritual energy? Ṛṣabhadeva says *mahāntas te sama-cittāḥ:* "The *mahātmās* are always equipoised, seeing everyone equally." As Lord Kṛṣṇa says in the *Bhagavad-gītā* (5.18):

vidyā-vinaya-sampanne brāhmaṇe gavi hastini
śuni caiva śva-pāke ca paṇḍitāḥ sama-darśinaḥ

"The humble sages, by virtue of true knowledge, see with equal vision a learned and gentle *brāhmaṇa,* a cow, an elephant, a dog, and a dog-eater [outcaste]." The *mahātmā* is equally disposed to everyone. He doesn't think, "He is American, so I shall be kind to him," or "He is Indian, so I shall be kind to him," or "He is black, so I shall be kind to him." No. He is kind to everyone.

Another quality of the *mahātmā* is that he is *praśāntā,* always very peaceful. Because he knows himself to be pure spirit, an eternal servant of Kṛṣṇa, he cannot be disturbed by any material condition. Also, he is *vimanyava,* free of anger, and *suhṛdaḥ,* a well-wisher for everyone. That is the vision of the *mahātmā.* He sees that people are suffering without God consciousness, without understanding their relationship with God, and so he tries to teach them. Therefore he has to be tolerant (*titikṣava*). When he tries to teach the people about Kṛṣṇa consciousness there will be so many insults, so many inconveniences. He has to tolerate them without becoming disturbed. In the Western countries Lord Jesus Christ perfectly showed this quality of tolerance. Because he was preaching about God consciousness, the state ordered that he be crucified. Still he prayed to God, "Please excuse them." So peacefulness, seeing everyone equally, freedom from anger, tolerance, mercy—these are the characteristics of a *mahātmā* or *sādhu,* a saintly person.

So we have to find such a person, associate with him, and serve him in full surrender. As Lord Kṛṣṇa says in the *Bhagavad-gītā* (4.34),

tad viddhi praṇipātena paripraśnena sevayā
upadekṣyanti te jñānaṁ jñāninas tattva-darśinaḥ

"Just try to learn the truth by approaching a spiritual master. Inquire from him submissively and render service unto him. The self-realized souls can impart knowledge unto you because they have seen the truth."

On the opposite side from service to the *sādhus* is *yoṣitāṁ saṅgi-saṅgam,* association with those who are too much attached to women. Actually, *yoṣitām* refers to anything enjoyable. There are so many things that attract us. Each sense has its own object of enjoyment. The eyes want to see beautiful forms. The tongue wants to enjoy very tasty food. The ears are attracted to nice singing. The nostrils are attracted to sweet fragrances. And the skin wants to touch soft things. All these are *yoṣitām,* enjoyable things, and people in general are attracted to all of them. They are going to the cinema, drinking wine, going to restaurants and clubs, and so on. And if we associate with persons who are attached to all these things for sense gratification, then the door to hell opens for us.

So you have to choose which door you will enter: one door leads to liberation from the entanglement of repeated birth and death and places us on the path back home, back to Godhead, and the other door, the door of sense gratification, leads to darkness (*adānta-gobhir viśatāṁ tamisram*). The more we indulge in sense gratification or associate with those who indulge in sense gratification, the deeper we go down into hellish life.

3: Achieving Unending Happiness

ye vā mayīśe kṛta-sauhṛdārthā
janeṣu dehambhara-vārtikeṣu
gṛheṣu jāyātmaja-rātimatsu
na prīti-yuktā yāvad-arthāś ca loke

Those who are interested in reviving Kṛṣṇa consciousness and increasing their love of Godhead do not like to do anything that is not related to Kṛṣṇa. They are not interested in mingling with people who are busy maintaining their bodies, eating, sleeping, mating, and defending. They are not attached to their homes, although they may be householders. Nor are they attached to wives, children, friends, or wealth. At the same time, they are not indifferent to the execution of their duties. Such people are interested in collecting only enough money to keep the body and soul together.

Śrīmad-Bhāgavatam 5.5.3

Whether he is an impersonalist or a devotee, one who is actually interested in advancing spiritually should not mingle with those who are simply interested in maintaining the body by means of the so-called advancement of civilization. Those who are interested in spiritual life should not be attached to homely comforts in the company of wife, children, friends, and so forth. Even if one is a householder and has to earn his livelihood, he should be satisfied by collecting only enough money to maintain body and soul together. One should not have more than that nor less than that. As indicated herein, a householder should endeavor to earn money for the execution of *bhakti-yoga,* or devotional service:

śravaṇaṁ kīrtanaṁ viṣṇoḥ smaraṇaṁ pāda-sevanam
arcanaṁ vandanaṁ dāsyaṁ sakhyam ātma-nivedanam

"The nine kinds of devotional service are hearing about Kṛṣṇa, chanting about Him, remembering Him, offering service to His lotus feet, offering Him worship in the temple, offering prayers to Him, working as His servant, making friendship with Him, and unreservedly surrendering to Him." (*Śrīmad-Bhāgavatam* 7.5.23) A householder should lead such a life that he gets a full opportunity to hear and chant about Kṛṣṇa. He should worship the Deity at home, observe festivals, and invite friends in and give them *prasādam,* food offered to Kṛṣṇa. A householder should earn money for this purpose, not for sense gratification.

Generally, however, people are interested only in maintaining their bodies. mahātmās*Śrīmad-Bhāgavatam* (2.1.3) says,

nidrayā hriyate naktaṁ vyavāyena ca vā vayaḥ
divā cārthehayā rājan kuṭumba-bharaṇena vā

At night they waste time by sleeping or indulging in sex, and during the daytime they are very busy trying to get some money. And as soon as they get money, they spend it to maintain their families. So where is the time for Kṛṣṇa consciousness? There is no time.

One should not be interested in mixing with those who are busy only with bodily affairs. One may be a householder, but one should be interested in devotional service to Kṛṣṇa, not simply in maintaining one's family. Such a householder *mahātmā* has no desire to associate with those who are interested only in bodily affairs. His only desire is to cultivate friendship with Kṛṣṇa (*ye vā mayīśe kṛta-sauhṛdārthā*). Then what about his family? Yes, he has his home, his wife, his children, and his means for earning money—but he's not very much interested. Officially he fulfills his family obligations, but his primary interest is Kṛṣṇa consciousness.

Of course, the householder *mahātmā* does not neglect his family responsibilities. He takes care of his children, his wife—

everything—but with a spirit of detachment: *anāsaktasya viṣayān yathārham upayuñjataḥ.* It is required that you educate your children and maintain your wife, but at the same time you should cultivate detachment. One should not think, "I shall sacrifice everything for my wife, children, and home." That is not a *mahātmā's* idea, because he knows that he cannot improve their destiny. Everyone has received a body with a destiny that he cannot change. So the scripture says, *tasyaiva hetoḥ prayateta kovido na labhyate yad bhramatām upary adhaḥ:* The wise person should try for advancement in Kṛṣṇa consciousness, not for material advancement. You may think, "If I work very hard, I shall improve my material position," but that is not possible. Your material position is already fixed. No one strives for distress, but distress comes automatically according to destiny. Similarly, if you have happiness in your destiny, it will come automatically, as the distress comes (*tal labhyate duḥkhavad anyataḥ sukham*). So don't be misled by material happiness and distress. They are already fixed. Simply try to advance in Kṛṣṇa consciousness and achieve unending transcendental happiness (*brahma-saukhyam tv anantam)*. That is your real business.

4: The Pain of Fleshly Pleasures

nūnaṁ pramattaḥ kurute vikarma
yad indriya-prītaya āpṛṇoti
na sādhu manye yata ātmano 'yam
asann api kleśada āsa dehaḥ

When a person considers sense gratification the aim of life, he certainly becomes mad after materialistic living and engages in all kinds of sinful activity. He does not know that due to his past misdeeds he has already received a body which, although temporary, is the cause of his misery. Actually the living entity should not have taken on a material body, but he has been awarded the material body for sense gratification. Therefore I think it not befitting an intelligent man to involve himself again in the activities of sense gratification, by which he perpetually gets material bodies one after another.

Śrīmad-Bhāgavatam 5.5.4

Begging, borrowing, and stealing to live for sense gratification is condemned in this verse because such consciousness leads one to a dark, hellish condition. The four sinful activities are illicit sex, meat-eating, intoxication, and gambling. These are the means by which one gets another material body, which is full of miseries. In the *Vedas* it is said: *asaṅgo hy ayaṁ puruṣaḥ.* The living entity is not really connected with this material world, but due to his tendency to enjoy the material senses, he is put into the material condition. One should perfect his life by associating with devotees. He should not become further implicated in the material body.

Here materialistic persons are described as *pramattaḥ,* "extremely mad or intoxicated." They're running here and there in their motorcars. From five o'clock in the morning or even earlier the main roads are full of motorcars. And what is the aim of such materialistic persons? *Yad indriya-prītaya āpṛṇoti:*

Their aim is to satisfy their senses. Eat, drink, be merry, and enjoy—that's all. Get money, go to the restaurant, go to the liquor shop, go to the prostitute house and the nightclub. They do not know anything more than *indriya-prīti,* sense gratification.

So they are all mad, and they are being implicated in so many sinful activities due to their desires for sense gratification. The result is that they get another material body after death. Everyone gets a certain type of body according to his sins and his specific desires for sense gratification. Otherwise, why are there so many varieties of life? Why is one soul born as a human being, another as a pig, another as a demigod, another as a tree, another as a fish? These varieties of life are all due to different desires for sense gratification and degrees of implication in sinful activities. Kṛṣṇa resides within the heart as the Supersoul, and he knows our desires and activities. As He says in the *Bhagavad-gītā* (18.61),

> *īśvaraḥ sarva-bhūtānāṁ hṛd-deśe 'rjuna tiṣṭhati*
> *bhrāmayan sarva-bhūtāni yantrārūḍhāni māyayā*

"The Īśvara, the Supreme Lord, is situated in everyone's heart as the Supersoul, overseeing the wanderings of the living entities in the material world." The materialist is always thinking, "If I would have acted like this, I would have gotten that opportunity, and then I would have enjoyed like this . . ." This kind of thinking is going on continually. And it is God's business—His thankless business—to note down, "All right, the rascal wants to enjoy like this, so I will give him such a facility." He's so merciful that He orders *māyā,* the material nature, "Give him such-and-such body so he can enjoy as he wants." Therefore we see so many varieties of bodies. They are all due to varieties of desire.

Unfortunately, all of these bodies are sources of misery (*kleśada*). Anyone who has a material body must suffer. Even the millionaire must suffer. There was once a very rich man in

Calcutta who could hardly eat. He had no appetite. He was served sumptuous food simply as a show, but he could not eat it. One day he saw a poor man passing on the street, carrying a fish and singing jubilantly. The rich gentleman said, "I am a rich man, but I have no appetite for all the many opulent foods that are served to me. Yet that poor man is thinking how he'll go home and cook his fish and eat it very nicely. He is so jubilant! If I would have been that poor man, at least I could have enjoyed some food." In spite of his becoming rich, he could not gratify his senses. His body was simply a source of misery.

So if you want to stop these varieties of material bodies, then you should give up all your nonsensical material desires. We already have a body that is a source of misery. Everyone has experience. No one can say, "My body never feels pain. I am perfect." That is not possible. As soon as you get a material body, it must be subjected to so many sufferings. Tribulations there must be. Therefore you should try to stop getting these material bodies. And to do this you must practice devotional service to Kṛṣṇa. Otherwise, you will continue on the path of birth and death. As Kṛṣṇa states in the *Bhagavad-gītā* (9.3),

aśraddadhānāḥ puruṣā dharmasyāsya parantapa
aprāpya māṁ nivartante mṛtyu-saṁsāra-vartmani

If you have no faith in the process of Kṛṣṇa consciousness you cannot attain Kṛṣṇa, and then you must continue on the path of birth and death—getting one body and again dying, getting another body and again dying.

In the modern age, education in these subjects is practically nil. It is very regrettable. But the information is there in the Vedic scriptures. And one who is intelligent will take advantage of this science, Kṛṣṇa consciousness, and mold his life accordingly so that he can stop this process of repeatedly accepting a body that is *kleśada,* the source of all miseries. That is the perfection of life.

5: Inquire into the Absolute

parābhavas tāvad abodha-jāto
yāvan na jijñāsata ātma-tattvam
yāvat kriyās tāvad idaṁ mano vai
karmātmakaṁ yena śarīra-bandhaḥ

As long as one does not inquire about the spiritual values of life, one is defeated and subjected to miseries arising from ignorance. Be it sinful or pious, karma has its resultant actions. If a person is engaged in any kind of karma, his mind is called karmātmaka, colored with fruitive activity. As long as the mind is impure, consciousness is unclear, and as long as one is absorbed in fruitive activity, he has to accept a material body.

Śrīmad-Bhāgavatam 5.5.5

Generally people think that one should act very piously in order to be relieved from misery, but this is not a fact. Even though one engages in pious activity and speculation, he is nonetheless defeated. His only aim should be emancipation from the clutches of *māyā* and all material activities. Speculative knowledge and pious activity do not solve the problems of material life. One should be inquisitive to understand his spiritual position. As stated in the *Bhagavad-gītā* (4.37):

yathaidhāṁsi samiddho 'gnir bhasmasāt kurute 'rjuna
jñānāgniḥ sarva-karmāṇi bhasmasāt kurute tathā

"As a blazing fire turns firewood to ashes, O Arjuna, so does the fire of knowledge burn to ashes all reactions to material activities."

Unless one understands the self and its activities, one has to be considered in material bondage. In *Śrīmad-Bhāgavatam* (10.2.32) it is said: *ye 'nye 'ravindākṣa vimukta-māninas tvayy asta-bhāvād aviśuddha-buddhayaḥ.* A person who doesn't have knowledge of devotional service may think himself liberated, but actually he is not. *Āruhya kṛcchreṇa paraṁ padaṁ tataḥ patanty adho 'nādṛta-yuṣmad-aṅghrayaḥ.* Such people may approach the impersonal Brahman effulgence, but they fall down again into material enjoyment because they have no knowledge of devotional service. As long as one is interested in *karma* and *jñāna,* he continues enduring the miseries of material life—birth, old age, disease, and death. *Karmīs* certainly take on one body after another. As far as *jñānīs* are concerned, unless they are promoted to the topmost understanding, they must return to the material world. As explained in the *Bhagavad-gītā* (7.19): *bahūnāṁ janmanām ante jñānavān māṁ prapadyate.* The point is to know Kṛṣṇa, Vāsudeva, as everything and surrender unto Him. *Karmīs* do not know this, but a devotee who is one hundred percent engaged in the devotional service of the Lord knows fully what is *karma* and *jñāna;* therefore a pure devotee is no longer interested in *karma* or *jñāna. Anyābhilāṣitā-śūnyaṁ jñāna-karmādy-anāvṛtam.* The real *bhakta* is untouched by any tinge of *karma* and *jñāna.* His only purpose in life is to serve the Lord. Therefore his mind is always engaged in thoughts of Kṛṣṇa, and he is free from bondage to a material body (*śarīra-bandhaḥ*). The material body is actually a great impediment to the soul, but in the modern so-called civilization there is no education on these matters.

In the state of bondage, whatever you do for your so-called material progress is ultimately defeated (*parābhava*). People are busily engaged throughout the day and night, thinking they are making material progress. But it is not progress: it is regression. This they do not know. Why? Because they never inquire into *ātma-tattva,* the spiritual values of life. Even big, big professors think that they have received their body by accident, and that as soon as the body is finished, everything is finished. That means they do not know the first lesson of *ātma-tattva—*

that the soul, or self, is eternal. And on the basis of this misconception they are inventing so many "isms"—communism, altruism, humanitarianism, etc.

Recently we talked with a medical man who was working on a cure for leprosy. That is good, but why should there be leprosy in the first place? Why is one man suffering from leprosy and another not suffering? Who is making this arrangement? These questions modern people do not ask, because they have become dull. And therefore whatever plans they make are baffled after some time (*parābhava*). They do not know what plans they should make for their ultimate benefit. For example, a child will think, "If I play like this, it will be very nice." So he engages in one type of play. And then he becomes dissatisfied and gives up that play and engages in another type of play. Out of ignorance (*abodha*), the child does not know where to find lasting happiness.

To dissipate this ignorance, one has to approach a person who is not *abodha* but *bodha,* full of knowledge. Such a person is called a *budhā,* wise man, because he knows the real goal of life and how to attain it. This word *budhā* is where Lord Buddha's name comes from. He understood everything. At first he was not a *budhā*—he was a prince, and he never came out of the palace. But one day he left the palace and saw an old man with a walking stick, walking with great difficulty. So he inquired from his servants: "What is this?" "This is an old man," they replied. "Everyone has to become like this." That was the inspiration for him to seek understanding. He inquired, "Why should he be like that? Why should one have to become an old man and be forced to walk with a stick?" So these inquiries made him a *budhā,* and he became Lord Buddha by meditation. Of course, that was his pastime. But he showed by example how inquisitiveness into the ultimate causes of suffering can lead one to proper knowledge. And where to get that proper knowledge? From a guru. The *Vedas* say, *tad-vijñānārthaṁ sa gurum evābhigacchet:* "If you want proper knowledge of the Absolute Truth, you must approach a bona fide guru."

People should be encouraged to inquire from the guru about the process for realizing the Absolute Truth: *sad-dharma pṛcchāt.* The student should be eager to know. It is not that one should accept the guru as a fashion. Nowadays many people do that. "Everyone has a dog, and everyone has a guru. So let me keep a guru." That is not the way to real understanding. One should be very inquisitive, but one should also serve the guru. As Kṛṣṇa says in the *Bhagavad-gītā* (4.34),

tad viddhi praṇipātena paripraśnena sevayā
upadekṣyanti te jñānaṁ jñāninas tattva-darśinaḥ

"Just try to learn the truth by approaching a spiritual master. Inquire from him submissively and render service unto him. The self-realized souls can impart knowledge unto you because they have seen the truth." You must be ready to serve the guru. Then you have the right to ask questions. First you must find a person to whom you can fully surrender (*praṇipātena*). Then you can inquire from him about *ātma-tattva,* spiritual science. And the inquiry should be accompanied by service. The more service you render to the guru, the more the truth is revealed.

yasya deve parā bhaktir yathā-deve tathā gurau
tasyaite kathitā hy arthāḥ prakāśante mahātmanaḥ

"Only unto those great souls who have unflinching devotion to the Lord and to the spiritual master is transcendental knowledge revealed."

6: Freedom Through Divine Love

evaṁ manaḥ karma-vaśaṁ prayuṅkte
avidyayātmany upadhīyamāne
prītir na yāvan mayi vāsudeve
na mucyate deha-yogena tāvat

When the living entity is covered by the mode of ignorance, he does not understand the individual living being and the supreme living being, and his mind is subjugated by fruitive activity. Therefore, until one has love for Lord Vāsudeva, who is none other than Myself [Ṛṣabhadeva], he is certainly not delivered from having to accept a material body again and again.

Śrīmad-Bhāgavatam 5.5.6

When the mind is polluted by fruitive activity, the living entity wants to be elevated from one material position to another. Generally everyone is involved in working hard day and night to improve his economic condition. Even when one understands the Vedic rituals, he becomes interested in promotion to heavenly planets, not knowing that one's real interest lies in returning home, back to Godhead. By acting on the platform of fruitive activity, one wanders throughout the universe in different species and forms. Unless he comes in contact with a devotee of the Lord, a guru, he does not become attached to the service of Lord Vāsudeva. Knowledge of Vāsudeva requires many births to understand. As confirmed in the *Bhagavad-gītā* (7.19): *vāsudevaḥ sarvam iti sa mahātmā sudurlabhaḥ.* After struggling for existence for many births one may take shelter at the lotus feet of Vāsudeva, Kṛṣṇa. When this happens, one actually becomes wise and surrenders unto Him. That is the only way to stop the repetition of birth and death. This is confirmed in the *Caitanya-caritāmṛta* (*Madhya* 19.151) in the instructions given by Śrī Caitanya Mahāprabhu to Śrīla Rūpa

Gosvāmī at Daśāśvamedha-ghāṭa.

brahmāṇḍa bhramite kona bhāgyavān jīva
guru-kṛṣṇa-prasāde pāya bhakti-latā-bīja

The living entity wanders throughout different planets in different forms and bodies, but if by chance he comes in contact with a bona fide spiritual master, by the grace of the spiritual master he receives Lord Kṛṣṇa's shelter, and his devotional life begins.

In material life the living entity's problem is contact with the material body. But nobody knows this. Especially these days people cannot understand that the material body is foreign to us and that we are entrapped within it and victimized by it. This is our real problem. But because of *avidyā,* ignorance, people do not know this. *Avidyā* is very strong when one is in the mode of passion (*rajo-guṇa*) or ignorance (*tamo-guṇa*). In the mode of goodness (*sattva-guṇa*) there is illumination. This means one has acquired brahminical qualifications. In that state one can understand, "I am not this body; I am different from it." For those in the mode of goodness, it is easier to advance in devotional life.

Human civilization should not drag someone in the mode of goodness down to the mode of ignorance. But the modern civilization does that. The allurements of the modern material civilization are so strong and so bad that even those who by previous pious activities are born in good families are being dragged down to sinful behavior. They are learning how to drink, how to eat meat, how to have illicit sex. These are the symptoms of the lowest type of ignorance. Real civilization means elevation. In other words, human civilization should be so arranged that everyone is gradually drawn to the mode of goodness, not dragged down to the mode of ignorance. But today the social, political, and economic arrangements are so bad that everyone is being dragged down to the mode of ignorance. This is not civilization. It is degradation. The aim of human life is to become liberated from the material body, and a civilization that elevates people to that platform is a real human civilization. Otherwise it is not civilization but animal life.

The Kṛṣṇa consciousness movement is attempting to bring human society to the platform of actual civilization. It is a very scientific movement. Here Lord Ṛṣabhadeva says, *prītir na yāvan mayi vāsudeve na mucyate deha-yogena tāvat:* "Until one develops love for Me, Vāsudeva, one will not be liberated from the material body." Since our problem is entrapment in the material body, we need a process by which we can develop love for Vāsudeva, or Kṛṣṇa, so we can be liberated from the body. That process is *bhakti,* or devotional service. One who follows the process of devotional service gradually comes to the platform of loving Kṛṣṇa. That is civilization—to bring one to the platform of loving Kṛṣṇa.

Real love means that one sees the beloved as everything (*vāsudevaṁ sarvam iti*). In this material world the closest thing we find to real love is a mother's love for her child. The mother loves the child so intensely that she is always anxious to take care of the child and her whole attention is on the child. From such an example we can understand something about real love, love for Kṛṣṇa. Material so-called love does not last, but nature dictates that you love your child, you love your husband, you love your wife, your country, your society. There are different varieties of love. But when that love is concentrated on Vāsudeva, Kṛṣṇa, it is the highest perfection of life.

You have to come to the stage of being firmly convinced that "Kṛṣṇa is my life." The highest perfection of this consciousness is displayed in Vṛndāvana, especially by the *gopīs*. Everyone in Vṛndāvana is attached to Kṛṣṇa—even the trees and plants, even the grains of sand. One cannot all of a sudden attain that highest stage of consciousness, but if one practices *bhakti-yoga* as we are teaching it, that stage will develop gradually. The proof is the success of this Kṛṣṇa consciousness movement. All over the world people who had never heard of Kṛṣṇa, who were in the lowest states of ignorance, are taking to Kṛṣṇa consciousness, and their love for Kṛṣṇa is gradually increasing. That is natural. As it is said in the *Caitanya-caritāmṛta* (*Madhya* 22.107):

nitya-siddha kṛṣṇa-prema 'sādhya' kabhu naya
śravaṇādi-śuddha-citte karaye udaya

"Pure love for Kṛṣṇa is eternally established in the hearts of the living entities. It is not something to be gained from another source. When the heart is purified by hearing and chanting about Kṛṣṇa, this love naturally awakens." Just as we are all eternal as living entities, so our devotion to Kṛṣṇa is eternal. Now it is simply covered by *avidyā,* ignorance. When we forget Kṛṣṇa, that is *avidyā,* and as soon as we take Kṛṣṇa as our life and soul, that is *vidyā. Avidyā* is darkness; *vidyā* is light. The Vedic injunction is *tamasi mā jyotir gama:* "Don't keep yourself in the darkness of ignorance; come to the light [*jyoti*] of Kṛṣṇa consciousness."

Ultimately that *jyoti* means love for Kṛṣṇa and the loving affairs of Kṛṣṇa in the spiritual world. That world is *jyotirmaya-dhāma,* Kṛṣṇa's self-effulgent abode. Just as in the sun there is no question of darkness, in the spiritual world there is also no question of darkness or ignorance. Everyone and everything there is in the state of *śuddha-sattva,* pure goodness. Not only goodness, but *pure* goodness. Here in this material world there are three modes—goodness, passion, and ignorance. None of these modes is pure: each is mixed with the others. And because there is a mixture, we see so many varieties of living beings. But we have to come to the platform of *śuddha-sattva,* pure goodness. The best process for this is hearing about Kṛṣṇa from authorized sources. The *Śrīmad-Bhāgavatam* (1.2.17) explains:

śṛṇvatāṁ sva-kathāḥ kṛṣṇaḥ puṇya-śravaṇa-kīrtanaḥ
hṛdy antaḥ stho hy abhadrāṇi vidhunoti suhṛt satām

"Śrī Kṛṣṇa, the Personality of Godhead, who is the Supersoul in everyone's heart and the benefactor of the truthful devotee, cleanses desire for material enjoyment from the heart of the devotee who has developed the urge to hear His messages, which are in themselves virtuous when properly heard and chanted." So if you seriously hear and chant about Kṛṣṇa, thinking "In this life I shall strive with great determination only to increase my love for Kṛṣṇa," it can be done. And as soon as you fully develop your love for Kṛṣṇa, there is no longer a chance of your being entrapped in a material body.

7: Don't Waste Time on Sense Pleasure

yadā na paśyaty ayathā guṇehāṁ
svārthe pramattaḥ sahasā vipaścit
gata-smṛtir vindati tatra tāpān
āsādya maithunyam agāram ajñaḥ

Even though one may be very learned and wise, he is mad if he does not understand that the endeavor for sense gratification is a useless waste of time. Being forgetful of his own interest, he tries to be happy in the material world, centering his interests on his home, which is based on sexual intercourse and which brings him all kinds of material miseries. In this way one is no better than a foolish animal.

Śrīmad-Bhāgavatam 5.5.7

In the lowest stage of devotional life, one is not an unalloyed devotee. *Anyābhilāṣitā-śūnyaṁ jñāna-karmādy-anāvṛtam:* to be an unalloyed devotee, one must be freed from all material desires and untouched by fruitive activity and speculative knowledge. On the lower platform, one may sometimes be interested in philosophical speculation with a tinge of devotion. However, at that stage one is still interested in sense gratification and is contaminated by the modes of material nature. The influence of *māyā* is so strong that even a person advanced in knowledge actually forgets that he is Kṛṣṇa's eternal servant. Therefore he remains satisfied in his householder life, which is centered on sexual intercourse. Conceding to a life of sex, he agrees to suffer all kinds of material miseries. Due to ignorance, one is thus bound by the chains of material laws.

Our real self-interest (*svārtha*) is to break these chains, but to understand this one has to be *vipaścit,* learned. Whether one is a fruitive worker, a speculator, a yogi, or a devotee, everyone is working for what he considers his self-interest. But for the devotees there is a little difference: they work for

Superself-interest, while others work for individual self-interest. The difference between working for self-interest and working for Superself-interest is the difference between lust and love, or *prema*. In the *Caitanya-caritāmṛta*, Kṛṣṇadāsa Kavirāja Gosvāmī has clearly explained this difference:

ātmendriya-prīti-vāñchā—tāre bali 'kāma'
kṛṣṇendriya-prīti-icchā dhare 'prema' nāma

"When one desires his personal sense gratification, that is *kāma,* or lust, and when one wants to satisfy the senses of Kṛṣṇa, that is *prema,* or love." (*Caitanya-caritāmṛta, Ādi-līlā* 4.165) The contrast between lust and love is shown in the *Bhagavad-gītā.* In the beginning of the *Bhagavad-gītā* Arjuna was thinking, "How can I possibly kill my brother, my nephews, my master, my teacher, my grandfather? I cannot do it; I refuse to fight." This calculation—in terms of the interest of his family and teacher—was for Arjuna's personal sense gratification. In other words, it was for his self-interest. But at the end of the *Bhagavad-gītā,* when Arjuna agreed to satisfy Kṛṣṇa by fighting, he was acting for Superself-interest. Arjuna had gone from *kāma* to *prema*.

For the materialistic person there are two kinds of self-interest. One is concentrated, and the other is extended. If you give a child a piece of cake, his immediate impulse is to eat it all himself, but if he is a little liberal he will give some to his friend. While the child is eating, his friend says, "Oh, you are eating cake? Give me some," "All right," the child replies, "you can take some." At first the child shows concentrated self-interest, and then extended self-interest. Another example is the big political leader. He is primarily interested in the welfare of himself and his family members—after all, self-preservation is the first law of nature—but he also works for the benefit of all members of the community, society, or country. But such extended self-interest can never be perfect, because there is always some fight between one community and another community, one society and another society, one nation and another nation. Only when that extended self-interest reaches up to Viṣṇu is it perfect. Then it is genuine self-interest, or Superself-interest.

Unfortunately, today people have no idea that serving the Supreme Lord, Viṣṇu or Kṛṣṇa, is their ultimate self-interest (*na te viduḥ svārtha-gatiṁ hi viṣṇum*). They think that if one extends his self-interest to his country, or even to all humanity, he will become a big man and people will honor him for his philanthropy. But that is not real philanthropy. Real philanthropy is serving Kṛṣṇa's interest. Otherwise it is all *kāma,* lust. Today's so-called philanthropy, altruism, and humanitarianism are all imperfect because they do not serve our ultimate self-interest. Again we can use the example of the cake. Suppose we pick up a nice piece of cake with our fingers. If the fingers think, "Now we have got it; we shall enjoy it ourselves," the cake will be spoiled. But if the fingers place it in the mouth, then their own interest will actually be served. As soon as the cake goes to the stomach, the energy is distributed not only to the fingers of the right hand but to those of the left hand also, and in fact to the whole body. Similarly, when one serves Kṛṣṇa's interest, everyone's interest is served because Kṛṣṇa is the root of everything. This law people do not know. Therefore here Lord Ṛṣabhadeva says, *svārthe pramattaḥ:* people do not know their real self-interest. Although everyone is trying individually, communally, and nationally to serve their self-interest, they do not know that their real self-interest lies in serving Kṛṣṇa.

Only in the human form of life can we understand our real self-interest. As Prahlāda Mahārāja says (7.6.1):

kaumāra ācaret prājño dharmān bhāgavatān iha
durlabhaṁ mānuṣaṁ janma tad apy adhruvam arthadam

"One who is sufficiently intelligent should use the human form of body from the very beginning of life—in other words, from the tender age of childhood—to practice the activities of devotional service, giving up all other engagements. The human body is most rarely achieved, and although temporary like other bodies, it is meaningful because in human life one can perform devotional service. Even a slight amount of sincere devotional service can give one complete perfection." As for physiological, anatomical, and even psychological construction, the human body is little different from the dog's. The dog has senses and we have senses, the dog has a mind and we have a mind, the dog has intelligence and we also have intelligence. The dog eats and we also eat, the dog sleeps and we also sleep. Similarly, if you cut an animal's body there will be blood, and if you cut a man's body there will also be blood. But the difference is that an animal cannot understand his real self-interest but a human being can. And if you act accordingly you can make your life successful. That is the special advantage of the human form of life. We should not waste it. As Narottama dāsa Ṭhākura has sung, taking the role of a conditioned soul:

hari hari biphale janama goṅāinu
manuṣya-janama pāiyā, rādhā-kṛṣṇa nā bhajiyā,
jāniyā śuniyā biṣa khāinu

"O Lord Kṛṣṇa, I have wasted my life. Although I have taken this rare human birth, I have not served Rādhā and Kṛṣṇa, and thus I have knowingly drunk poison." Sometimes we may take poison unknowingly—food poison or some other poison—but if one takes poison *knowingly,* that means he's killing himself. Similarly, in this human form of life, if we do not come to the understanding that without Kṛṣṇa consciousness our life is wasted, we are simply taking poison. Then our life is spoiled. We will be put into a miserable condition birth after birth. That is nature's way. You cannot escape the stringent laws of material nature. As Kṛṣṇa states in the *Bhagavad-gītā* (9.3):

aśraddadhānāḥ puruṣā dharmasyāsya parantapa
aprāpya māṁ nivartante mṛtyu-saṁsāra-vartmani

"Those who are not faithful in this devotional service cannot attain Me, O conqueror of enemies. Therefore they return to the path of birth and death in this material world." On account of false prestige, false knowledge, and false education, people think they are independent of God, that they can do whatever they like. We have to give up this mentality; otherwise we will have to continue in the miserable cycle of birth and death because we have forgotten our real position.

Here Lord Ṛṣabhadeva states that the main reason people foolishly forget their position as servants of Kṛṣṇa and suffer material pangs is sex: *maithunyam agāram ajñaḥ.* We see people working so hard day and night. Sometimes they start for their business or office as early as five in the morning and do not return until ten o'clock at night. Why are they working so hard? For the pleasure of sex indulgence, that's all. Their main happiness is enjoying sexual intercourse at night. Prahlāda Mahārāja states that the pleasures a materialistic householder enjoys, centered on sex, are very insignificant (*tuccham*). Indeed, such a person's home becomes a prison house (*agāra*), and he remains shackled by the iron chains of sex. Only a fool would accept this lowest class of happiness as the aim of life. So don't be foolish; be intelligent and understand that your real self-interest lies in worshiping Kṛṣṇa.

8: Sex Is the Main Cause of Bondage

puṁsaḥ striyā mithunī-bhāvam etaṁ
tayor mitho hṛdaya-granthim āhuḥ
ato gṛha-kṣetra-sutāpta-vittair
janasya moho 'yam ahaṁ mameti

The attraction between male and female is the basic principle of material existence. On the basis of this misconception, which ties together the hearts of the male and female, one becomes attracted to his body, home, property, children, relatives, and wealth. In this way one increases life's illusions and thinks in terms of "I and mine."

Śrīmad-Bhāgavatam 5.5.8

Sex serves as the natural attraction between man and woman, and when they are married their relationship becomes more involved. Due to the entangling relationship between man and woman, there is a sense of illusion whereby one thinks, "This man is my husband" or "This woman is my wife." This is called *hṛdaya-granthi,* "the hard knot in the heart." This knot is very difficult to undo, even though a man and woman separate either for the principles of *varṇāśrama* or simply to get a divorce. In any case, the man always thinks of the woman, and the woman always thinks of the man. Thus a person becomes materially attached to family, property, and children, although all of these are temporary. The possessor unfortunately identifies with his property and wealth. Sometimes, even after renunciation, one becomes attached to a temple or to the few things that constitute the property of a *sannyāsī,* but such attachment is not as strong as family attachment. The attachment to the family is the strongest illusion. In the *Satya-saṁhitā,* it is stated:

brahmādyā yājñavalkyādyā mucyante strī-sahāyinaḥ
bodhyante kecanaiteṣāṁ viśeṣam ca vido viduḥ

Sometimes it is found among exalted personalities like Lord Brahmā that the wife and children are not a cause of bondage. On the contrary, the wife actually helps further spiritual life and liberation. Nonetheless, most people are bound by the knots of the marital relationship, and consequently they forget their relationship with Kṛṣṇa.

So sex attraction is the beginning of the illusion summarized in the phrase *ahaṁ mameti:* "I am my body, and everything in relationship with my body is mine." A man searches after a woman, and a woman searches after a man, and when they unite for sex the material illusion becomes very strong. This is nature's arrangement for keeping the conditioned soul under her stringent laws. As it is said,

kṛṣṇa-bahirmukha haiyā bhoga-vāñchā kare
nikaṭa-stha māyā tāre jāpaṭiyā dhare

"As soon as one becomes inimical to Kṛṣṇa and desires sense gratification, he is immediately struck down by the illusory energy of the Lord." This is just like breaking the laws of the state. We have practical experience that as soon as we refuse to obey the state laws we immediately become criminals and are subjected to prosecution and imprisonment. Just as you cannot defy the state laws without being punished by the government, you cannot defy Kṛṣṇa's laws without being punished by the laws of nature. But because we are in illusion, we think our effort to diminish this punishment is advancement of civilization.

The whole material world is based on the attraction between male and female. This principle is working not only in human society but among the birds, beasts, aquatics, insects—everywhere. You will find that as soon as a male pigeon sees a female pigeon, the male immediately begins canvassing: "Please come, let us unite." This is nature's way. Therefore, in human society one has to understand by Vedic knowledge, by education, that we are bound up within this material world due to sex attraction. Both the male and the female want to be the enjoyer. Nobody is thinking "I shall be enjoyed." Everyone is thinking, "I shall enjoy." Nobody wants to be predominated; everyone wants to be the predominator. This is illusion.

The Kṛṣṇa consciousness movement is teaching everyone to give up this idea of being the predominator and learn how to be predominated by the Supreme Lord, Kṛṣṇa. Just the opposite of the illusory materialistic idea. Kṛṣṇa comes personally and says, "Why are you trying to be the predominator? That is not possible. I am the predominator. Just surrender to Me and you will be happy." *Sarva-dharmān parityajya mām ekaṁ śaraṇaṁ vraja.* But if you artificially want to be the predominator, then immediately Kṛṣṇa's illusory energy (*māyā*) is there to entrap you.

We should know that this inclination to be the enjoyer and predominator is the cause of our bondage within this material world. We should know that we are spirit (*ahaṁ brahmāsmi*), without birth or death. Then we should ask, "If as spirit I do not take birth or die, why am I subjected to the sufferings of this material world such as birth and death? Why have I been put into this condition?" That is intelligence. We are not meant to be conditioned, because we are part and parcel of Kṛṣṇa. Kṛṣṇa is free of all conditioning, and in our natural state we are also free. We may be very small particles of Kṛṣṇa, but just as a gold particle has all the qualities of the mass of gold in the gold mine, so we have all of Kṛṣṇa's qualities in minute degree. We can acquire knowledge of all these things when we follow the instruction of the *Vedānta-sūtra: athāto brahma jijñāsā.* "Now, therefore, one should inquire into the Absolute Truth."

Unless one inquires into the Absolute Truth and learns how to make a complete solution to the problems of life, one's life is no better than an animal's. In other words, if one remains satisfied in a miserable condition of life, then he is nothing but an animal. Animals cannot understand why they're suffering.

When animals are being taken to the slaughterhouse, if one animal enters the slaughterhouse, then every animal will enter easily. They do not understand that they are entering to be slaughtered. This is illusion.

So, here Lord Ṛṣabhadeva is teaching that sex is the cause of the greatest illusion for human beings. Therefore, traditional Vedic education taught young boys the value of celibacy, *brahmacarya.* "Don't become entangled with sex life. It is not good. Better to remain celibate. You will be happy." But if one is unable to remain celibate, one may take a wife and live as a gentleman, a regulated householder, or *gṛhastha,* not like cats and dogs. A life of unrestricted sex is not human civilization.

There are many rules and regulations for *gṛhastha* life. *Gṛhastha* life does not permit you to have sex whenever you like. No: once in a month, when conception is most likely; and if the wife is pregnant, then no more sex. That is *gṛhastha* life. Not that a man and woman simply unite and live like animals. That is not *gṛhastha* life but *gṛhamedhi* life. A *gṛhamedhi* is one who does not follow the rules and regulations of married life. He thinks that the pleasure he derives from his wife, children, and home is everything. But a genuine *gṛhastha* is as good as a *sannyāsī* (renunciant). That is why a householder who follows the regulative principles is said to be in the *gṛhastha-āśrama.* An *āśrama* is a place where spiritual life is cultivated. What is the difference between the *gṛhastha-āśrama* and an ordinary home? In an ordinary home one does not follow any regulative principles because one's only purpose is to enjoy sex, family life, and so on, but in the *gṛhastha-āśrama* one leads a regulated life because one's real purpose is self-realization, the development of Kṛṣṇa consciousness.

So, as far as possible we should avoid entanglement in sex life. This avoidance is real austerity (*tapasya*). Lord Ṛṣabhadeva began his instructions by recommending austerity: *tapo divyaṁ putrakā yena sattvam śuddhyet.* "O my sons, perform transcendental austerity, by which your existence will be purified." Such austerity begins with celibacy (*tapasā brahmacāryeṇa*). But Kṛṣṇa consciousness is so nice that if one accepts its principles very seriously, then anyone—man or woman, married or unmarried—can remain very happy with Kṛṣṇa as one's master, one's son, one's friend, one's husband, or one's lover. In this way, as we advance in Kṛṣṇa consciousness, we can save ourselves from the galaxy of illusion known as this material world, in which there is simply suffering after suffering after suffering.

9: Untie the Knot of Attachment

yadā mano-hṛdaya-granthir asya
karmānubaddho dṛḍha āślatheta
tadā janaḥ samparivartate 'smād
muktaḥ paraṁ yāty atihāya hetum

When the strong knot in the heart of a person implicated in material life due to the results of past action is slackened, one turns away from his attachment to home, wife, and children. In this way, one gives up the basic principle of illusion [I and mine] and becomes liberated. Thus one goes to the transcendental world.

Śrīmad-Bhāgavatam 5.5.9

When, by associating with sadhus and engaging in devotional service, one is gradually freed from the material conception due to knowledge, practice, and detachment, the knot of attachment in the heart is slackened. Thus one can get freed from conditioned life and become eligible to return home, back to Godhead.

Here Lord Ṛṣabhadeva is describing the process of liberation. Liberation means no more material life, and the basic principle of material life is sex. Therefore Vedic civilization is based on training people how to become free from sex desire. The great emperor Yāmunācārya described his own experience in this regard:

yad-avadhi mama cetaḥ kṛṣṇa-pādāravinde
nava-nava-rasa-dhāmany udyataṁ rantum āsīt
tad-avadhi bata nārī-saṅgame smaryamāne
bhavati mukha-vikāraḥ suṣṭhu niṣṭhīvanaṁ ca

"Ever since I have given my mind and heart to the loving service of the lotus feet of Lord Kṛṣṇa, I have increased my transcendental, blissful life by rendering such service, and thus when I happen to think of sex life, I consider it so abominable that I spit at the thought." This kind of distaste for sex is a sign of advancement in Kṛṣṇa conscious life.

The four pillars of degradation are illicit sex, meat-eating, intoxication, and gambling. Therefore we forbid our students to indulge in these practices. If you want to make progress in Kṛṣṇa consciousness, you must give these up. When Śrī Caitanya Mahāprabhu delivered Jagāi and Mādhāi, who were addicted to all these practices, the Lord made this condition: "If you promise to give up these four principles of sinful life, I will accept you. Never mind what you have done in the past. Every man is sinful, more or less; there is no doubt about it. That is not a disqualification. But if you agree to give them up now, then immediately you are liberated." Liberation is not very difficult. You can obtain it in a minute, provided you want to take it. Kṛṣṇa promises this in the *Bhagavad-gītā* (18.66):

sarva-dharmān parityajya mām ekaṁ śaraṇaṁ vraja
ahaṁ tvāṁ sarva-pāpebhyo mokṣayiṣyāmi mā śucaḥ

"Abandon all varieties of religion and just surrender unto Me. I shall deliver you from all sinful reactions. Do not fear." If you are free from the reactions of sinful life, you are liberated. In other words, you are liberated if you get shelter at the lotus feet of Kṛṣṇa and do not act in such a way that you again fall down into sin. The *Śrīmad-Bhāgavatam* defines liberation as *hitvānyathā-rūpaṁ svarūpeṇa vyavasthitiḥ*—giving up our false identification with our gross and subtle bodies and being situated in our *svarūpa. Svarūpa* means our original, constitutional position. Lord Caitanya explains: *jīvera svarūpa haya kṛṣṇera nitya-dāsa:* "The constitutional position of the living entity is to be an eternal servant of Kṛṣṇa." And as soon as we place ourselves in our original, constitutional position, we are liberated.

Kṛṣṇa describes our constitutional position very simply in the *Bhagavad-gītā: man-manā bhava mad-bhaktaḥ.* "Always think of Me and be ready to serve Me. That's all." The word *bhakta* ("devotee") implies *bhakti* ("devotional service") and Bhagavān, the Supreme Personality of Godhead. So, when one engages in devotional service to the Supreme Personality of Godhead, Lord Kṛṣṇa, one is situated in one's constitutional position and is liberated. This means the hard knot of attachment in the heart is slackened.

One has to understand that he is becoming more and more entangled by material attachments, beginning with sex desire, and that these attachments are engaging him more and more in fruitive activity. When we understand this and try to get free from this business, we become eligible for going back home, back to Godhead. Here Ṛṣabhadeva uses the word *samparivartate,* meaning one has to turn away from the cause of bondage—sex, wife, home, etc.—and turn back toward Kṛṣṇa. That is liberation.

10: The Path to the Highest Pleasure

haṁse gurau mayi bhaktyānuvṛtyā
vitṛṣṇayā dvandva-titikṣayā ca
sarvatra jantor vyasanāvagatyā
jijñāsayā tapasehā-nivṛttyā

mat-karmabhir mat-kathayā ca nityaṁ
mad-deva-saṅgād guṇa-kīrtanān me
nirvaira-sāmyopaśamena putrā
jihāsayā deha-gehātma-buddheḥ

adhyātma-yogena vivikta-sevayā
prāṇendriyātmābhijayena sadhryak
sac-chraddhayā brahmacaryeṇa śaśvad
asampramādena yamena vācām

sarvatra mad-bhāva-vicakṣaṇena
jñānena vijñāna-virājitena
yogena dhṛty-udyama-sattva-yukto
liṅgaṁ vyapohet kuśalo 'ham-ākhyam

O My sons, you should accept a highly elevated paramahaṁsa, a spiritually advanced spiritual master. In this way, you should place your faith and love in Me, the Supreme Personality of Godhead. You should detest sense gratification and tolerate the duality of pleasure and pain, which are like the seasonal changes of summer and winter. Try to realize the miserable condition of living entities, who are miserable even in the higher planetary systems. Philosophically inquire about the truth. Then undergo all kinds of austerities and penances for the sake of devotional service. Give up the endeavor for sense enjoyment and engage in the service of the Lord. Listen to discussions about the Supreme Personality of Godhead, and always associate with devotees. Chant about and glorify the

Supreme Lord, and look upon everyone equally on the spiritual platform. Give up enmity and subdue anger and lamentation. Abandon identifying the self with the body and the home, and practice reading the revealed scriptures. Live in a secluded place and practice the process by which you can completely control your life air, mind, and senses. Have full faith in the revealed scriptures, the Vedic literatures, and always observe celibacy. Perform your prescribed duties and avoid unnecessary talks. Always thinking of the Supreme Personality of Godhead, acquire knowledge from the right source. Thus practicing bhakti-yoga, you will patiently and enthusiastically be elevated in knowledge and will be able to give up the false ego.

Śrīmad-Bhāgavatam 5.5.10–13

In these four verses, Ṛṣabhadeva tells His sons how they can become free from false ego in material, conditioned life. One gradually becomes liberated by practicing as mentioned above. All these prescribed methods enable one to give up the material body (*liṅgaṁ vyapohet*) and be situated in his original spiritual body. First of all one has to accept a bona fide spiritual master. This is advocated by Śrīla Rūpa Gosvāmī in his *Bhakti-rasāmṛta-sindhu: śrī-guru-pādāśrayaḥ.* To be freed from the entanglement of the material world, one has to approach a spiritual master. *Tad-vijñānārthaṁ sa gurum evābhigacchet* (*Muṇḍaka Upaniṣad* 1.2.12). By questioning the spiritual master and by serving him, one can advance in spiritual life. When one engages in devotional service, naturally the attraction for personal comfort—for eating, sleeping, and dressing—is reduced. When one associates with devotees, a spiritual standard is maintained. The word *mad-deva-saṅgāt* ("association with My devotees") is very important. There are many so-called religions devoted to the worship of various demigods, but here good association means association with one who simply accepts Kṛṣṇa as his worshipable Deity.

Another important item is *dvandva-titikṣā* ("tolerance of material dualities"). As long as one is situated in the material world, there must be pleasure and pain arising from the material body. As Kṛṣṇa advises in the *Bhagavad-gītā, tāṁs titikṣasva bhārata.* One has to learn how to tolerate the temporary pains and pleasures of this material world. One must also be detached from his family and practice celibacy. Sex with one's wife according to the scriptural injunctions is also accepted as *brahmacarya* (celibacy), but illicit sex is opposed to religious principles, and it hampers advancement in spiritual consciousness. Another important word is *vijñāna-virājita.* Everything should be done very scientifically and consciously. One should be a realized soul. In this way, one can give up the entanglement of material bondage.

As Śrī Madhvācārya points out, the sum and substance of these four *ślokas* is that one should refrain from acting out of a desire for sense gratification and should instead always engage in the Lord's loving service. In other words, *bhakti-yoga* is the acknowledged path of liberation. Śrīla Madhvācārya quotes from the *Adhyātma:*

ātmano 'vihitaṁ karma varjayitvānya-karmaṇaḥ
kāmasya ca parityāgo nirīhety āhur uttamāḥ

One should perform activities only for the benefit of the soul; any other activity should be given up. When a person is situated in this way, he is said to be desireless. Actually a living entity cannot be totally desireless, but when he desires the benefit of the soul and nothing else, he is said to be desireless.

Spiritual knowledge is *jñāna-vijñāna-samanvitam.* When one is fully equipped with *jñāna* and *vijñāna,* he is perfect. *Jñāna* means that one understands the Supreme Personality of Godhead, Viṣṇu, to be the Supreme Being. *Vijñāna* refers to the activities that liberate one from the ignorance of material existence. As stated in *Śrīmad-Bhāgavatam* (2.9.31): *jñānaṁ parama-guhyaṁ me yad vijñāna-samanvitam.* Knowledge of the Supreme Lord is very confidential, and the supreme knowledge by which one understands Him furthers the liberation of all living entities. This knowledge is *vijñāna.* As Lord Kṛṣṇa confirms in the *Bhagavad-gītā* (4.9):

janma karma ca me divyam evaṁ yo vetti tattvataḥ
tyaktvā dehaṁ punar janma naiti mām eti so 'rjuna

"One who knows the transcendental nature of My appearance and activities does not, upon leaving the body, take his birth again in this material world, but attains My eternal abode, O Arjuna."

In Text 9 Lord Ṛṣabhadeva recommended that one slacken the knots of attachment in the heart, and the items listed in these verses are the means by which one can do this. Unfortunately, in the modern world almost everyone is busy from morning till late at night increasing those attachments. Working in big, big factories day and night, one shift after another—this unnecessarily severe hard work (*ugra-karma*) has become a most conspicuous feature of modern civilization. We have seen such *ugra-karma* in Detroit. In the assembly plants where they manufacture Ford motorcars, one man is simply putting on the wheels of the motorcar. He has a huge stock of wheels nearby. And somebody else is putting on the tires. He has a huge stock of tires. There are so many motorcar parts—three thousand parts. So there are big, big factories elsewhere where men are working day and night to manufacture the different parts of the motorcar. And ultimately the parts are sent to the factory in Detroit where they assemble one car after another, and people are using a huge quantity of cars. After working day and night in the factories, people try to pacify themselves by intoxication and illicit sex. All this *ugra-karma* keeps one bound up by unlimited material attachments.

Despite all this *ugra-karma,* however, people are not happy.

They do not know that happiness cannot be had from *ugra-karma.* Therefore here Lord Ṛṣabhadeva says that one of the principles of advancement is *sarvatra jantor vyasanāvagatyā,* seeing that in the material world there is misery everywhere, even on higher planets. As Kṛṣṇa says in the *Bhagavad-gītā, ā-brahma-bhuvanāl lokāḥ punar āvartino 'rjuna:* "From the highest planet down to the lowest, all are places of misery." And also, *duḥkhālayam aśāṣvatam*: "This material world is a place of misery where life is temporary."

So, we should know that although we are trying to improve our material condition in so many ways, it is ultimately impossible to do so. If a poor man works very hard and acquires a great amount of wealth, that does not mean he is free from the dangerous conditions of life, because the threefold miseries are present everywhere. These are miseries pertaining to the body and mind, miseries caused by other living entities, and miseries brought on by the forces of nature. And of course there are always the miseries of birth, old age, disease, and death.

All these miseries are caused by the material body, whose root is the false ego. This false ego can be given up if we take up the practices Lord Ṛṣabhadeva describes here: *liṅgaṁ vyapohet kuśalo 'ham-ākhyam.* The first practice is surrendering to a highly advanced spiritual master (*haṁse gurau mayi bhaktyānuvṛtyā*). This is the beginning of real religion. If you do not get a qualified guru, then everything is bogus. But if by good fortune you get the association of a qualified guru, then you can receive the seed of the creeper of devotion. As Lord Caitanya says, *guru-kṛṣṇa-prasāde pāya bhakti-latā-bīja:* "By the mercy of both the spiritual master and Kṛṣṇa, the fortunate soul receives within his heart the seed of the creeper of devotion." Therefore here Ṛṣabhadeva, who is an incarnation of Kṛṣṇa, says *haṁse gurau mayi bhaktyānuvṛtyā:* "One must render devotional service first to the spiritual master and then to Me." You cannot jump over the spiritual master and go to Kṛṣṇa. Some rascals say, "Well, I know Kṛṣṇa. I shall go to

Kṛṣṇa directly, without a guru." No, that is not possible. First of all guru, then Kṛṣṇa. And if one actually follows the instructions given by the guru and the scriptures, then one's strong desire to enjoy this material world will be slackened and one's liberation from material miseries is assured.

11: Attaining All Perfection

karmāśayaṁ hṛdaya-granthi-bandham
avidyayāsāditam apramattaḥ
anena yogena yathopadeśaṁ
samyag vyapohyoparameta yogāt

As I have advised you, My dear sons, you should act accordingly. Be very careful. By these means you will be freed from the ignorance of the desire for fruitive activity, and the knot of bondage in the heart will be completely severed. For further advancement, you should also give up the means. That is, you should not become attached to the process of liberation itself.

Śrīmad-Bhāgavatam 5.5.14

The process of liberation is *brahma jijñāsā,* the search for the Absolute Truth. Generally *brahma jijñāsā* is called *neti neti,* the process by which one analyzes existence to search out the Absolute Truth. This method continues as long as one is not situated in his spiritual life. Spiritual life is *brahma-bhūta,* the self-realized state. In the words of the *Bhagavad-gītā* (18.54):

brahma-bhūtaḥ prasannātmā na śocati na kāṅkṣati
samaḥ sarveṣu bhūteṣu mad-bhaktiṁ labhate parām

"One who is thus transcendentally situated at once realizes the Supreme Brahman and becomes fully joyful. He never laments nor desires to have anything; he is equally disposed to every living entity. In that state, he attains pure devotional service unto Me."

The idea is to enter into the *parā bhakti,* the transcendental devotional service of the Supreme Lord. To attain this, one must analyze one's existence, but when one is actually engaged in devotional service he should not bother seeking out knowledge. By simply engaging in devotional service undeviatingly, one will always remain in the liberated condition.

māṁ ca yo 'vyabhicāreṇa bhakti-yogena sevate
sa guṇān samatītyaitān brahma-bhūyāya kalpate
Bhagavad-gītā 14.26

The unflinching execution of devotional service automatically places one on the transcendental platform, called the *brahma-bhūta* stage. Another important feature in this connection is *anena yogena yathopadeśam.* The instructions received from the spiritual master must be followed immediately. One should not deviate from or surpass the instructions of the spiritual master. One should not be simply intent on consulting books but should simultaneously execute the spiritual master's order (*yathopadeśam*). Mystic power should be achieved to enable one to give up the material conception, but when one actually engages in devotional service, one does not need to practice the mystic yoga system. The point is that one can give up the practice of yoga but devotional service cannot be given up. As stated in the *Śrīmad-Bhāgavatam* (1.7.10):

ātmārāmāś ca munayo nirgranthā apy urukrame
kurvanty ahaitukīṁ bhaktim itthaṁ-bhūta-guṇo hariḥ

Even those who are liberated [*ātmārāma*] must always engage in devotional service. One may give up the practice of yoga when one is self-realized, but at no stage can one give up devotional service. All other activities for self-realization, including yoga and philosophical speculation, may be given up, but devotional service must be retained at all times.

Devotional service will free us from *karmāśayam,* the desire for fruitive activity. As long as our mind is absorbed in fruitive activity, there is no question of becoming free from bondage to the material body (*karmātmakaṁ yena śarīra-bandhaḥ*). The whole purpose of human life is to free the spirit soul from bondage to the body and thus from the suffering caused by the repetition of birth and death. Everyone is trying to become happy by working hard and enjoying the results—not only here on earth but also on other planets, even up to the highest planet, Brahmaloka. But this process simply increases our bondage to the material body. In Texts 10 through 13 Lord Ṛṣabhadeva explained the process of devotional service, by which one can gradually become free from this bondage.

Devotional service is a science; it is not sentiment. Therefore we have to understand it from authorized sources of Vedic knowledge. Such knowledge is not based on our imperfect senses, and so in the Vedic knowledge there is no mistake, cheating, or illusion. Everything is perfect. This is real science—perfect knowledge. Not "perhaps," "it may be"—that is not science but theory.

To know the science of devotional service, one has to approach a perfect teacher (*tad-vijñānārthaṁ sa gurum evābhigacchet*). In Text 10 Lord Ṛṣabhadeva confirms that the first step in devotional service is *haṁse gurau mayi bhaktyānuvṛtyā:* "One should surrender to a highly elevated spiritual master and in this way render devotional service to Me, the Supreme Personality of Godhead." The word *mayi,* "unto Me, the Supreme Personality of Godhead," is significant. This indicates that the guru is as good as the Supreme Lord because he does not deviate from the instructions of the Lord. That is the primary characteristic of the guru: he does not manufacture something new. No, he teaches the same thing that Kṛṣṇa taught five thousand years ago in the *Bhagavad-gītā.* And even when Kṛṣṇa spoke it then it was not new. In the Fourth Chapter of the *Bhagavad-gītā* (4.1) Kṛṣṇa says to Arjuna, *sa evāyaṁ mayā te 'dya yogaḥ proktaḥ purātanaḥ:* "The same science of yoga I instructed to the sun-god millions of years ago I am instructing today to you." It is not that because time has passed the instruction must be changed. This is nonsense. There cannot be something new in the matter of the science of the Absolute Truth. Everything is established. Millions of years ago the sun rose on the eastern horizon, and still it is rising in the east. It is not that now the sun is rising on the western or northern horizon. Similarly, Vedic knowledge is eternally established. It cannot be changed under any circumstance. What was true millions of years ago is true now. And to know that truth, one has to approach a bona fide spiritual master.

Two of the most important steps in devotional service given by Lord Ṛṣabhadeva are *mat-karmabhiḥ,* "working for Me," and *mat-kathayā ca nityam,* "always hearing and chanting words concerning Me." The word *nityam,* "always," is very important here. One should not attend classes in *Śrīmad-Bhāgavatam* for seven or ten days a year and the other 355 days go to the stock market and simply inquire about the price of this share or that share. No, you have to hear the *Bhāgavatam* daily in the association of devotees (*mad-deva-saṅgāt*), not in the association of fruitive workers or mental speculators. That will not help us.

Another important item in devotional service is *jihāsayā deha-gehātma-buddhi:* By executing devotional service one should develop detachment from family life. In the *Bhāgavatam* (11.2.42) it is said, *bhaktiḥ pareśānubhavo viraktir anyatra ca:* "By the practice of *bhakti-yoga* one feels the transcendental pleasure of serving the Lord, experiences His presence, and feels detachment from everything else." That is *bhakti-yoga.* Everyone can test his progress on the path of devotional service by asking himself, "How much have I become detached from worldly affection? How much am I still thinking 'This is my body, this is my country, this is my society, this is my wife, these are my children'?" We have to give up these illusory attachments. If we are not able to give up worldly attachment, then we cannot make any progress. One has to come to understand *ahaṁ brahmāsmi:* "I am not this body, I am not this mind, I am not this intelligence. I am pure spirit [*brahman*], part and parcel of Kṛṣṇa, the Supreme Brahman."

If we practice devotional service according to the instructions given here in the *Bhāgavatam* and in other bona fide scriptures (*śāstras*), we will be successful and become liberated. But without scripture, it is not possible. As Kṛṣṇa says in the *Bhagavad-gītā* (16.23), *yaḥ śāstra-vidhim utsṛjya vartate kāma-kārataḥ na sa siddhim avāpnoti:* "If you give up the instructions of scripture and act according to your whims, then there is no question of perfection." And Rūpa Gosvāmī confirms this in his *Bhakti-rasāmṛta-sindhu* (1.2.101):

śruti-smṛti-purāṇādi- pañcarātra-vidhiṁ vinā
aikāntikī harer bhaktir utpātāyaiva kalpate

"Devotional service of the Lord that ignores the authorized Vedic literatures like the *Upaniṣads, Purāṇas,* and *Nārada-pañcarātra* is simply an unnecessary disturbance in society." There are so many religious practices that have been invented. For example, the scriptures prescribe the chanting of the Hare Kṛṣṇa mantra, but people have invented so many ways of chanting. If you chant Rāma Rāma Rāma, Rādhe Rādhe Rādhe, Kṛṣṇa Kṛṣṇa Kṛṣṇa, that is also chanting the holy name, but you have to follow the scripture. The scripture says chant Hare Kṛṣṇa, Hare Kṛṣṇa, Kṛṣṇa Kṛṣṇa, Hare Hare/ Hare Rāma, Hare Rāma, Rāma Rāma, Hare Hare. You have to accept that. Not that you chant *nitāi-gaura rādhe-śyāma, hare kṛṣṇa hare rāma.* No. What is the value of your invention? You are not perfect. You cannot invent a new mantra and be successful. Simply follow the recommendations of scripture and you will attain all perfection.

Kṛṣṇa Consciousness at Home

by Mahātmā dāsa

In *Spiritual Yoga* Śrīla Prabhupāda makes it clear how important it is for everyone to practice Kṛṣṇa consciousness, devotional service to Lord Kṛṣṇa. Of course, living in the association of Kṛṣṇa's devotees in a temple or ashram makes it easier to practice devotional service. But if you're determined, you can follow at home the teachings of Kṛṣṇa consciousness and thus convert your home into a temple.

Spiritual life, like material life, means practical activity. The difference is that whereas we perform material activities for the benefit of ourselves or those we consider ours, we perform spiritual activities for the benefit of Lord Kṛṣṇa, under the guidance of the scriptures and the spiritual master. The key is to accept the guidance of the scripture and the guru. Kṛṣṇa declares in the *Bhagavad-gītā* that a person can achieve neither happiness nor the supreme destination of life—going back to Godhead, back to Lord Kṛṣṇa—if he or she does not follow the injunctions of the scriptures. And *how* to follow the scriptural rules by engaging in practical service to the Lord—that is explained by a bona fide spiritual master. Without following the instructions of a spiritual master who is in an authorized chain of disciplic succession coming from Kṛṣṇa Himself, we cannot make spiritual progress. The practices outlined here are the timeless practices of *bhakti-yoga* as given by the foremost spiritual master and exponent of Kṛṣṇa consciousness in our time, His Divine Grace A. C. Bhaktivedanta Swami Prabhupāda, founder-*ācārya* of the International Society for Krishna Consciousness (ISKCON).

The purpose of spiritual knowledge is to bring us closer to God, or Kṛṣṇa. Kṛṣṇa says in the *Bhagavad-gītā* (18.55), *bhaktyā māṁ abhijānāti:* "I can be known only by devotional service." Knowledge guides us in proper action. Spiritual knowledge directs us to satisfy the desires of Kṛṣṇa through practical engagements in His loving service. Without practical application, theoretical knowledge is of little value.

Spiritual knowledge is meant to direct us in all aspects of life. We should endeavor, therefore, to organize our lives in such a way as to follow Kṛṣṇa's teachings as far as possible. We should try to do our best, to do more than is simply convenient. Then it will be possible for us to rise to the transcendental plane of Kṛṣṇa consciousness, even while living far from a temple.

Chanting the Hare Kṛṣṇa Mantra

The first principle in devotional service is to chant the Hare Kṛṣṇa *mahā-mantra* (*mahā* means "great"; *mantra* means "sound that liberates the mind from ignorance"):

Hare Kṛṣṇa, Hare Kṛṣṇa, Kṛṣṇa Kṛṣṇa, Hare Hare
Hare Rāma, Hare Rāma, Rāma Rāma, Hare Hare

You should chant these holy names of the Lord as much as possible—anywhere and at any time—but it is also very helpful to set a specific time of the day to regularly chant. Early morning hours are ideal.

The chanting can be done in two ways: singing the mantra, called *kīrtana* (usually done in a group), and saying the mantra to oneself, called *japa* (which literally means "to speak softly"). Concentrate on hearing the sound of the holy names. As you chant, pronounce the names clearly and distinctly, addressing Kṛṣṇa in a prayerful mood. When your mind wanders, bring it back to the sound of the Lord's names. Chanting is a prayer to Kṛṣṇa that means "O energy of the Lord [Hare], O all-attractive Lord [Kṛṣṇa], O Supreme Enjoyer [Rāma], please engage me in Your service." The more attentively and sincerely you chant these names of God, the more spiritual progress you will make. Since God is all-powerful and all-merciful, He has kindly made it very easy for us to chant His names, and He has also invested all His powers in them. Therefore the names of God and God Himself are identical. This means that when we chant the holy names of Kṛṣṇa and Rāma we are directly associating with God and being purified. Therefore we should always try to chant with devotion and reverence. The Vedic literature states that Lord Kṛṣṇa is personally dancing on your tongue when you chant His holy name.

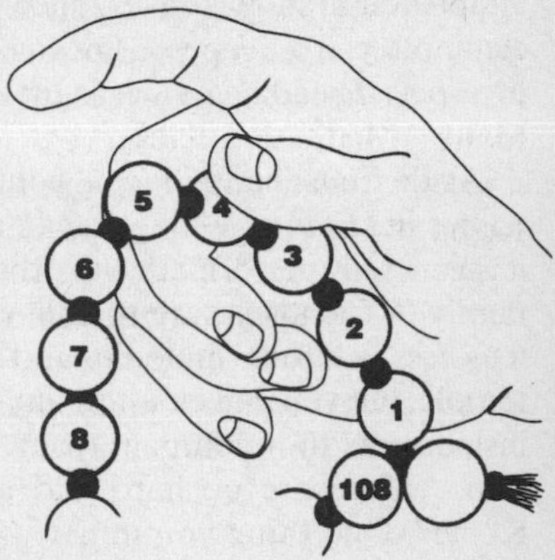

When you chant alone, it is best to chant on *japa* beads (call the mailorder branch of the Bhaktivedanta Book Trust, at 1-800-927-4152). This not only helps you fix your attention on the holy name, but it also helps you count the number of times you chant the mantra daily. Each strand of *japa* beads contains 108 small beads and one large bead, the head bead. Begin on a bead next to the head bead and gently roll it between the thumb and middle finger of your right hand as you chant the full Hare Kṛṣṇa mantra. Then move to the next bead and repeat the process. In this way, chant on each of the 108 beads until you reach the head bead again. This is one round of *japa*. Then, without chanting on the head bead, reverse the beads and start your second round on the last bead you chanted on.

Initiated devotees vow before the spiritual master to chant at least sixteen rounds of the Hare Kṛṣṇa mantra daily. But even if you can chant only one round a day, the principle is that once you commit yourself to chanting that round, you should try to complete it every day without fail. When you feel you can chant more, then increase the minimum number of rounds you chant each day—but don't fall below that number. You can chant more than your fixed number, but you should maintain a set minimum each day. (Please note that the beads are sacred and therefore should never touch the ground or be put in an unclean place. To keep your beads clean, it's best to carry them in a special bead bag, such as the one that comes as part of the Mantra Meditation Kit.)

Aside from chanting *japa,* you can also sing the Lord's holy names in *kīrtana*. While you can perform *kīrtana* individually, it is generally performed with others. A melodious *kīrtana* with family or friends is sure to enliven everyone. ISKCON devotees use traditional melodies and instruments, especially in the temple, but you can chant to any melody and use any musical instruments to accompany your chanting. As Lord Caitanya said, "There are no hard and fast rules for chanting Hare Kṛṣṇa." One thing you might want to do, however, is order some *kīrtana* and *japa* audiotapes or CDs (see ads).

Setting Up Your Altar

You will likely find that your *japa* and *kīrtana* are especially effective when done before an altar. Lord Kṛṣṇa and His pure devotees are so kind that they allow us to worship them even through their pictures. It is something like mailing a letter: You cannot mail a letter by placing it in just any box; you must use the mailbox authorized by the government. Similarly, we cannot imagine a picture of God and worship that, but we can worship the authorized picture of God, and Kṛṣṇa accepts our worship through that picture.

Setting up an altar at home means receiving the Lord and His pure devotees as your most honored guests. Where should you set up the altar? Well, how would you seat a guest? An ideal place would be clean, well lit, and free from drafts and household disturbances. Your guest, of course, would need a comfortable chair, but for the picture of Kṛṣṇa's form a wall shelf, a mantelpiece, a corner table, or the top shelf of a bookcase will do. You wouldn't seat a guest in your home and then

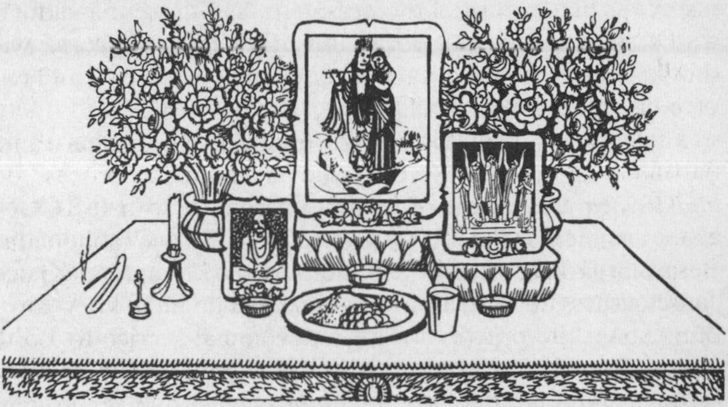

ignore him; you'd provide a place for yourself to sit, too, where you could comfortably face him and enjoy his company. So don't make your altar inaccessible.

What do you need for an altar? Here are the essentials:

1. A picture of Śrīla Prabhupāda.
2. A picture of Lord Caitanya and His associates.
3. A picture of Śrī Śrī Rādhā-Kṛṣṇa.

In addition, you may want an altar cloth, water cups (one for each picture), candles with holders, a special plate for offering food, a small bell, incense, an incense holder, and fresh flowers, which you may offer in vases or simply place beforeeach picture. If you're interested in more elaborate Deity worship, ask any of the ISKCON devotees or get in touch with the BBT (call 1-800-927-4152).

The first person we worship on the altar is the spiritual master. The spiritual master is not God. Only God is God. But because the spiritual master is His dearmost servant, God has empowered him, and therefore he deserves the same respect as that given to God. He links the disciple with God and teaches him the process of *bhakti-yoga.* He is God's ambassador to the material world. When a president sends an ambassador to a foreign country, the ambassador receives the same respect as that accorded the president, and the ambassador's words are as authoritative as the president's. Similarly, we should respect the spiritual master as we would God, and revere his words as we would His.

There are two main kinds of gurus: the instructing guru and the initiating guru. Everyone who takes up the process of *bhakti-yoga* as a result of coming in contact with ISKCON owes an immense debt of gratitude to Śrīla Prabhupāda. Before Śrīla Prabhupāda left India in 1965 to spread Kṛṣṇa consciousness abroad, almost no one outside India knew anything about the practice of pure devotional service to Lord Kṛṣṇa. Therefore, everyone who has learned of the process through his books, his *Back to Godhead* magazine, recordings of his words, or contact with his followers should offer respect to Śrīla Prabhupāda. As the founder and spiritual guide of the International Society for Krishna Consciousness, he is the instructing guru of us all.

As you progress in *bhakti-yoga,* you may eventually want to accept initiation. Before he left this world in 1977, Śrīla Prabhupāda encouraged his qualified disciples to carry on his work by initiating disciples of their own in accordance with his instructions. At present there are many spiritual masters in ISKCON. To learn how you can get spiritual guidance from them, ask a devotee at your nearby temple, or write to one of the ISKCON centers listed at the end of this book.

The second picture on your altar should be one of the *pañca-tattva,* Lord Caitanya and His four leading associates. Lord Caitanya is the incarnation of God for this age. He is Kṛṣṇa Himself, descended in the form of His own devotee to teach us how to surrender to Him, specifically by chanting His holy names and performing other activities of *bhakti-yoga.* Lord Caitanya is the most merciful incarnation, for He makes it easy for anyone to attain love of God through the chanting of the Hare Kṛṣṇa *mantra.*

And of course your altar should have a picture of the

Supreme Personality of Godhead, Lord Śrī Kṛṣṇa, with His eternal consort, Śrīmatī Rādhārāṇī. Śrīmatī Rādhārāṇī is Kṛṣṇa's spiritual potency. She is devotional service personified, and devotees always take shelter of Her to learn how to serve Kṛṣṇa.

You can arrange the pictures in a triangle, with the picture of Śrīla Prabhupāda on the left, the picture of Lord Caitanya and His associates on the right, and the picture of Rādhā and Kṛṣṇa, which, if possible, should be slightly larger than the others, on a small raised platform behind and in the center. Or you can hang the picture of Rādhā and Kṛṣṇa on the wall above.

Carefully clean the altar each morning. Cleanliness is essential in Deity worship. Remember, you wouldn't neglect to clean the room of an important guest, and when you establish an altar you invite Kṛṣṇa and His pure devotees to reside as the most exalted guests in your home. If you have water cups, rinse them out and fill them with fresh water daily. Then place them conveniently close to the pictures. You should remove flowers in vases as soon as they're slightly wilted, or daily if you've offered them at the base of the pictures. You should offer fresh incense at least once a day, and, if possible, light candles and place them near the pictures when you're chanting before the altar.

Please try the things we've suggested so far. It's very simple, really: If you try to love God, you'll gradually realize how much He loves you. That's the essence of *bhakti-yoga.*

Prasādam: How to Eat Spiritually

By His immense transcendental energies, Kṛṣṇa can actually convert matter into spirit. If we place an iron rod in a fire, before long the rod becomes red hot and acts just like fire. In the same way, food prepared for and offered to Kṛṣṇa with love and devotion becomes completely spiritualized. Such food is called Kṛṣṇa *prasādam,* which means "the mercy of Lord Kṛṣṇa."

Eating *prasādam* is a fundamental practice of *bhakti-yoga.*

In other forms of yoga one must artificially repress the senses, but the *bhakti-yogī* can engage his or her senses in a variety of pleasing spiritual activities, such as tasting delicious food offered to Lord Kṛṣṇa. In this way the senses gradually become spiritualized and bring the devotee more and more transcendental pleasure by being engaged in devotional service. Such spiritual pleasure far surpasses any material experience.

Lord Caitanya said of *prasādam,* "Everyone has tasted these foods before. However, now that they have been prepared for Kṛṣṇa and offered to Him with devotion, these foods have acquired extraordinary tastes and uncommon fragrances. Just taste them and see the difference in the experience! Apart from the taste, even the fragrance pleases the mind and makes one forget any other fragrance. Therefore, it should be understood that the spiritual nectar of Kṛṣṇa's lips must have touched these ordinary foods and imparted to them all their transcendental qualities."

Eating only food offered to Kṛṣṇa is the perfection of vegetarianism. In itself, being a vegetarian is not enough; after all, even pigeons and monkeys are vegetarians. But when we go beyond vegetarianism to a diet of *prasādam,* our eating becomes helpful in achieving the goal of human life—reawakening the soul's original relationship with God. In the *Bhagavad-gītā* Lord Kṛṣṇa says that unless one eats only food that has been offered to him in sacrifice, one will suffer the reactions of karma.

How to Prepare and Offer Prasādam

As you walk down the supermarket aisles selecting the foods you will offer to Kṛṣṇa, you need to know what is offerable and what is not. In the *Bhagavad-gītā,* Lord Kṛṣṇa states, "If one offers Me with love and devotion a leaf, a flower, a fruit, or water, I will accept it." From this verse it is understood that we can offer Kṛṣṇa foods prepared from milk products, vegetables, fruits, nuts, and grains. (Call 1-800-927-4152 for Hare Kṛṣṇa cookbooks.) Meat, fish, and eggs are not offerable. And a few vegetarian items are also forbidden—garlic and onions, for example, which are in the mode of darkness. (Hing, or asafetida, is a tasty substitute for them in cooking and is available at most Indian groceries and ISKCON temple stores.) Nor can you offer to Kṛṣṇa coffee or tea that contain caffeine. If you like these beverages, purchase caffeine-free coffee and herbal teas.

While shopping, be aware that you may find meat, fish, and egg products mixed with other foods; so be sure to read labels carefully. For instance, some brands of yogurt and sour cream contain gelatin, a substance made from the horns, hooves, and bones of slaughtered animals. Also, make sure the cheese you buy contains no animal rennet, an enzyme from the stomach tissues of slaughtered calves. Most hard cheese sold in America contains this rennet, so be careful about any cheese you can't verify as being free from animal rennet.

Also avoid foods cooked by nondevotees. According to the subtle laws of nature, the cook acts upon the food not only physically but mentally as well. Food thus becomes an agent for subtle influences on your consciousness. The principle is the same as that at work with a painting: a painting is not simply a collection of strokes on a canvas but an expression of the artist's state of mind, which affects the viewer. So if you eat food cooked by nondevotees—employees working in a factory, for example—then you're sure to absorb a dose of materialism and karma. So as far as possible use only fresh, natural ingredients.

In preparing food, cleanliness is the most important principle. Nothing impure should be offered to God; so keep your kitchen very clean. Always wash your hands thoroughly before entering the kitchen. While preparing food, do not taste it, for you are cooking the meal not for yourself but for the pleasure of Kṛṣṇa. Arrange portions of the food on dinnerware kept especially for this purpose; no one but the Lord should eat from these dishes. The easiest way to offer food is simply to pray, "My dear Lord Kṛṣṇa, please accept this food," and to chant each of the following prayers three times while ringing a bell (see the Sanskrit Pronunciation Guide on page 62):

1. Prayer to Śrīla Prabhupāda:

nama oṁ viṣṇu-pādāya kṛṣṇa-preṣṭhāya bhū-tale
śrīmate bhaktivedānta- svāminn iti nāmine

namas te sārasvate deve gaura-vāṇī-pracāriṇe
nirviśeṣa-śūnyavādi- pāścātya-deśa-tāriṇe

"I offer my respectful obeisances unto His Divine Grace A. C. Bhaktivedanta Swami Prabhupāda, who is very dear to Lord Kṛṣṇa on this earth, having taken shelter at His lotus feet. Our respectful obeisances are unto you, O spiritual master, servant of Bhaktisiddhānta Sarasvatī Gosvāmī. You are kindly preaching the message of Lord Caitanyadeva and delivering the Western countries, which are filled with impersonalism and voidism."

2. Prayer to Lord Caitanya:

namo mahā-vadānyāya kṛṣṇa-prema-pradāya te
kṛṣṇāya kṛṣṇa-caitanya- nāmne gaura-tviṣe namaḥ

"O most munificent incarnation! You are Kṛṣṇa Himself appearing as Śrī Kṛṣṇa Caitanya Mahāprabhu. You have assumed the golden color of Śrīmatī Rādhārāṇī, and You are widely distributing pure love of Kṛṣṇa. We offer our respectful obeisances unto You."

3. Prayer to Lord Kṛṣṇa:

namo brahmaṇya-devāya go-brāhmaṇa-hitāya ca
jagad-dhitāya kṛṣṇāya govindāya namo namaḥ

"I offer my respectful obeisances unto Lord Kṛṣṇa, who is the worshipable Deity for all *brāhmaṇas,* the well-wisher of the cows and the *brāhmaṇas,* and the benefactor of the whole world. I offer my repeated obeisances to the Personality of Godhead, known as Kṛṣṇa and Govinda."

Remember that the real purpose of preparing and offering food to the Lord is to show your devotion and gratitude to Him. Kṛṣṇa accepts your devotion, not the physical offering itself. God is complete in Himself—He doesn't need anything—but out of His immense kindness He allows us to offer food to Him so that we can develop our love for Him.

After offering the food to the Lord, wait at least five minutes for Him to partake of the preparations. Then you should transfer the food from the special dinnerware and wash the dishes and utensils you used for the offering. Now you and any guests may eat the *prasādam.* While you eat, try to appreciate the spiritual value of the food. Remember that because Kṛṣṇa has accepted it, it is nondifferent from Him, and therefore by eating it you will become purified.

Everything you offer on your altar becomes *prasādam,* the mercy of the Lord. Flowers, incense, the water, the food—everything you offer for the Lord's pleasure becomes spiritualized. The Lord enters into the offerings, and thus the remnants are nondifferent from Him. So you should not only deeply respect the things you've offered, but you should distribute them to others as well. Distribution of *prasādam* is an essential part of Deity worship.

Everyday Life: The Four Regulative Principles

Anyone serious about progressing in Kṛṣṇa consciousness must try to avoid the following four sinful activities:

1. Eating meat, fish, or eggs. These foods are saturated with the modes of passion and ignorance and therefore cannot be offered to the Lord. A person who eats these foods participates

in a conspiracy of violence against helpless animals and thus stops his spiritual progress dead in its tracks.

2. Gambling. Gambling invariably puts one into anxiety and fuels greed, envy, and anger.

3. The use of intoxicants. Drugs, alcohol, and tobacco, as well as any drinks or foods containing caffeine, cloud the mind, overstimulate the senses, and make it impossible to understand or follow the principles of *bhakti-yoga*.

4. Illicit sex. This is sex outside of marriage or sex in marriage for any purpose other than procreation. Sex for pleasure compels one to identify with the body and takes one far from Kṛṣṇa consciousness. The scriptures teach that sex is the most powerful force binding us to the material world. Anyone serious about advancing in Kṛṣṇa consciousness should minimize sex or eliminate it entirely.

Engagement in Practical Devotional Service

Everyone must do some kind of work, but if you work only for yourself you must accept the karmic reactions of that work. As Lord Kṛṣṇa says in the *Bhagavad-gītā* (3.9), "Work done as a sacrifice for Viṣṇu [Kṛṣṇa] has to be performed. Otherwise work binds one to the material world."

You needn't change your occupation, except if you're now engaged in a sinful job such as working as a butcher or bartender. If you're a writer, write for Kṛṣṇa; if you're an artist, create for Kṛṣṇa; if you're a secretary, type for Kṛṣṇa. You may also directly help the temple in your spare time, and you should sacrifice some of the fruits of your work by contributing a portion of your earnings to help maintain the temple and propagate Kṛṣṇa consciousness. Some devotees living outside the temple buy Hare Kṛṣṇa literature and distribute it to their friends and associates, or they engage in a variety of services at the temple. There is also a wide network of devotees who gather in each other's homes for chanting, worship, and study.

Write to your local temple or the Society's secretary to learn of any such programs near you.

Additional Devotional Principles

There are many more devotional practices that can help you become Kṛṣṇa conscious. Here are two vital ones:

Studying Hare Kṛṣṇa literature. Śrīla Prabhupāda, the founder-*ācārya* of ISKCON, dedicated much of his time to writing books such as the *Bhagavad-gītā As It Is* and *Śrīmad-Bhāgavatam,* both of which are quoted extensively in *Spiritual Yoga*. Hearing the words—or reading the writings—of a realized spiritual master is an essential spiritual practice. So try to set aside some time every day to read Śrīla Prabhupāda's books. You can get a free catalog of available books and other media from the BBT.

Associating with devotees. Śrīla Prabhupāda established the Hare Kṛṣṇa movement to give people in general the chance to associate with devotees of the Lord. This is the best way to gain faith in the process of Kṛṣṇa consciousness and become enthusiastic in devotional service. Conversely, maintaining intimate connections with nondevotees slows one's spiritual progress. So try to visit the Hare Kṛṣṇa center nearest you as often as possible.

In Closing

The beauty of Kṛṣṇa consciousness is that you can take as much as you're ready for. Kṛṣṇa Himself promises in the *Bhagavad-gītā* (2.40), "There is no loss or diminution in this endeavor, and even a little advancement on this path protects one from the most fearful type of danger." So bring Kṛṣṇa into your daily life, and we guarantee you'll feel the benefit.

Hare Kṛṣṇa!

Sanskrit Pronunciation Guide

The system of transliteration used in this book conforms to a system that scholars have accepted to indicate the pronunciation of each sound in the Sanskrit language.

The short vowel **a** is pronounced like the **u** in b**u**t, long **ā** like the **a** in f**a**r. Short **i** is pronounced as in p**i**n, long **ī** as in p**i**que, short **u** as in p**u**ll, and long **ū** as in r**u**le. The vowel **ṛ** is pronounced like the **ri** in **ri**m, **e** like the **ey** in th**ey**, **o** like the **o** in g**o**, **ai** like the **ai** in **ai**sle, and **au** like the **ow** in h**ow**. The *anusvāra* (**ṁ**) is pronounced like the **n** in the French word *bo***n**, and *visarga* (**ḥ**) is pronounced as a final **h** sound. At the end of a couplet, **aḥ** is pronounced **aha**, and **iḥ** is pronounced **ihi**.

The guttural consonants—**k, kh, g, gh,** and **ṅ**—are pronounced from the throat in much the same manner as in English. **K** is pronounced as in **k**ite, **kh** as in Ec**kh**art, **g** as in **g**ive, **gh** as in di**g h**ard, and **ṅ** as in si**ng.**

The palatal consonants—**c, ch, j, jh,** and **ñ**—are pronounced with the tongue touching the firm ridge behind the teeth. **C** is pronounced as in **ch**air, **ch** as in staun**ch-h**eart, **j** as in **j**oy, **jh** as in he**dgeh**og, and **ñ** as in ca**ny**on.

The cerebral consonants—**ṭ, ṭh, ḍ, ḍh,** and **ṇ**—are pronounced with the tip of the tongue turned up and drawn back against the dome of the palate. **Ṭ** is pronounced as in **t**ub, **ṭh** as in ligh**t-h**eart, **ḍ** as in **d**ove, **ḍh** as in re**d-h**ot, and **ṇ** as in **n**ut. The dental consonants—**t, th, d, dh,** and **n**—are pronounced in the same manner as the cerebrals, but with the forepart of the tongue against the teeth.

The labial consonants—**p, ph, b, bh,** and **m**—are pronounced with the lips. **P** is pronounced as in **p**ine, **ph** as in u**ph**ill, **b** as in **b**ird, **bh** as in ru**b-h**ard, and **m** as in **m**other.

The semivowels—**y, r, l,** and **v**—are pronounced as in **y**es, **r**un, **l**ight, and **v**ine respectively. The sibilants—**ś, ṣ,** and **s**—are pronounced, respectively, as in the German word **s***prechen* and the English words **sh**ine and **s**un. The letter **h** is pronounced as in **h**ome.

Glossary

A

Absolute Truth—the ultimate source of all energies.

Arjuna—one of the five Pāṇḍava brothers. Kṛṣṇa became his chariot driver and spoke the *Bhagavad-gītā* to him.

B

Bhagavad-gītā—a seven-hundred-verse record of a conversation between Lord Kṛṣṇa and His disciple Arjuna, recorded in the *Mahābhārata.*

Bhakti-yoga—the system of cultivation of *bhakti,* or pure devotional service to God, which is untinged by sense gratification or philosophical speculation.

Brahmā—the first created living being and secondary creator of the material universe.

Brahman—the impersonal, all-pervasive aspect of the Supreme.

Brāhmaṇa—a member of the intellectual, priestly class; a person wise in Vedic knowledge, fixed in goodness, and knowledgeable of Brahman, the Absolute Truth.

C

Caitanya-caritāmṛta—the foremost biography of Lord Caitanya Mahāprabhu. Written in Bengali and Sanskrit in the late sixteenth century by Śrīla Kṛṣṇadāsa Kavirāja Gosvāmī, it brilliantly presents the Lord's pastimes and teachings.

Caitanya Mahāprabhu (1486–1534)—Lord Kṛṣṇa in the aspect of His own devotee. He appeared in Navadvīpa, West Bengal, and inaugurated the congregational chanting of the holy names of the Lord to teach pure love of God.

D

Demigods—universal controllers and residents of the higher planets.

F

False ego—the conception that "I am this material body, mind, or intelligence."

G

Gopīs—Kṛṣṇa's cowherd girlfriends, who are His most surrendered and confidential devotees.

Guru—spiritual master.

I

Impersonalist—one who adheres to the philosophy that everything is one and that the Absolute Truth is not a person.

J

Jñāna—knowledge. Material *jñāna* does not go beyond the material body. Transcendental *jñāna* discriminates between matter and spirit. Perfect *jñāna* is knowledge of the body, the soul, and the Supreme Lord.

Jñānī—one engaged in the cultivation of knowledge, especially by philosophical speculation.

K

Karma—any material action that will incur a subsequent reaction.

Karmīs—fruitive workers.

Kṛṣṇa—the Supreme Personality of Godhead, i.e., the original, two-armed form of the Supreme Lord, who is the origin of all expansions.

M

Madhvācārya—a great devotee scholar and teacher who lived in India during the thirteenth century A.D.

Mahābhārata—an important and famous historical Vedic scripture.

Mahātmā—literally a "great soul," who understands that Kṛṣṇa is everything and who therefore surrenders unto Him.

Mantra—a transcendental sound or Vedic hymn.

N

Nārada-pañcarātra—Nārada Muni's book on the processes of Deity worship and mantra meditation.

Narottama dāsa Ṭhākura—a renowned sixteenth-century Vaiṣṇava spiritual master in the disciplic succession from Lord Śrī Caitanya Mahāprabhu. He is famous for writing many devotional songs.

P

Padma Purāṇa—one of the eighteen *Purāṇas,* or Vedic historical scriptures.

Parabrahman—the Supreme Brahman, the Personality of Godhead, Śrī Kṛṣṇa.

Param Brahma—*See:* Parabrahman.

Prahlāda Mahārāja—a great devotee of Lord Kṛṣṇa who was persecuted by his atheistic father, Hiraṇyakaśipu, but was always protected by the Lord and ultimately saved by Him in the form of Nṛsiṁhadeva, the Lord's half-man, half-lion incarnation.

Purāṇas—the eighteen historical supplements to the *Vedas.*

R

Ṛṣabhadeva—an incarnation of the Supreme Lord as a devotee king who, after instructing his sons in spiritual life, renounced His kingdom for a life of austerity.

Rūpa Gosvāmī—chief of the Six Gosvāmīs of Vṛndāvana, who were empowered by Lord Caitanya Mahāprabhu to establish and distribute the philosophy of Kṛṣṇa consciousness.

S

Sannyāsī—one in the renounced order, the fourth stage of Vedic spiritual life in the Vedic system of *varṇāśrama-dharma.* A *sannyāsī* is free from family relationships and dedicates all his activities to Kṛṣṇa.

Śloka—a Sanskrit verse.

Śrīmad-Bhāgavatam—the foremost of the eighteen *Purāṇas.* The complete science of God, it establishes the supreme position of Lord Kṛṣṇa.

Supersoul—the localized aspect of the Supreme Lord, residing in the heart of each embodied living entity and pervading all of material nature.

U

Upaniṣads—one-hundred-eight Sanskrit treatises that embody the philosophy of the *Vedas.*

V

Vaiṣṇava—a devotee of Viṣṇu, or Kṛṣṇa.

Varṇāśrama-dharma—the system of four social and four spiritual orders established in the Vedic scriptures and discussed by Śrī Kṛṣṇa in the *Bhagavad-gītā.*

Vāsudeva—the Supreme Lord, Kṛṣṇa, son of Vasudeva and proprietor of everything, material and spiritual.

Vedānta-sūtra—Śrīla Vyāsadeva's conclusive summary of Vedic philosophical knowledge, written in aphorisms.

Vedas—the four original scriptures (*Ṛg, Sāma, Atharva,* and *Yajur).*

Vedic—pertaining to a culture in which all aspects of human life are under the guidance of the *Vedas.*

Vijñāna—the practical realization of spiritual knowledge.

Viṣṇu Purāṇa—a scripture describing the glories of Lord Viṣṇu. *See also: Purāṇas.*

Vṛndāvana—Kṛṣṇa's eternal abode, where He fully manifests His quality of sweetness; the village on this earth where He enacted His childhood pastimes five thousand years ago.

Yāmunācārya—a great Vaiṣṇava spiritual master and author in the Śrī-sampradāya, one of the important disciplic lines of Vaiṣṇavas.

The International Society for Krishna Consciousness
Founder-Ācārya: His Divine Grace A.C. Bhaktivedanta Swami Prabhupāda

CENTERS AROUND THE WORLD

(Partial List)

NORTH AMERICA

CANADA

Calgary, Alberta — 313 Fourth Street N.E., T2E 3S3/ Tel. (403) 265-3302/ Fax: (403) 547-0795/E-mail: vamanstones@shaw.ca

Edmonton, Alberta — 9353 35th Ave., T6E 5R5/ Tel. (403) 439-9999

Montreal, Quebec — 1626 Pie IX Boulevard, H1V 2C5/ Tel. & fax: (514) 521-1301/ E-mail: temple@iskconmontreal.com

♦ **Ottawa, Ontario** — 212 Somerset St. E., K1N 6V4/ Tel. (613) 565-6544/ Fax: (613) 565-2575/ E-mail: iskconottawa@sympatico.ca

Regina, Saskatchewan — 1279 Retallack St., S4T 2H8/ Tel. (306) 525-1640

♦ **Toronto, Ontario** — 243 Avenue Rd., M5R 2J6/ Tel. (416) 922-5415/ Fax: (416) 922-1021/ E-mail: toronto@iskcon.net

♦ **Vancouver, B.C.** — 5462 S.E. Marine Dr., Burnaby V5J 3G8/ Tel. (604) 433-9728/ Fax: (604) 648-8715/ E-mail: jaygo@telus.net; Govinda's Bookstore & Cafe/ Tel. (604) 433-7100 or 1-888-433-8722/ E-mail: jaygo@telus.net

RURAL COMMUNITY

Ashcroft, B.C. — Saranagati Dhama (mail: P.O. Box 99, V0K 1A0, attn: Uttama Devi Dasi)/ Tel. (250) 453-2397/ Fax: (250) 453-2622 [attn: (250) 453-2397]/ E-mail: uttamadd@yahoo.com

U.S.A.

Alachua, Florida — 17306 N.W. 112th Blvd., 32615 (mail: P.O. Box 819, 32616)/ Tel. (386) 462-2017/ Fax: (386) 462-3468/ E-mail: alachua@pamho.net

♦ **Atlanta, Georgia** — 1287 South Ponce de Leon Ave. N.E., 30306/ Tel. & fax: (404) 377-8680/ E-mail: bala108@earthlink.net

Austin, Texas — 10700 Jonwood Way, 78753/ Tel. (512) 835-2121/ Fax: (512) 835-8479/ E-mail: harekrishna@swbell.net

Baltimore, Maryland — 200 Bloomsbury Ave., Catonsville 21228/ Tel. & fax: (410) 744-1624/ E-mail: sporecki@earthlink.net

Berkeley, California — 2334 Stuart Street, 94705/ Tel. (510) 649-8619/ Fax: (510) 841-7619/ E-mail: rasaraja@bvinst.edu

Boise, Idaho — 1615 Martha St., 83706/ Tel. (208) 344-4274/ E-mail: boise_temple@yahoo.com

Boston, Massachusetts — 72 Commonwealth Ave., 02116/ Tel. (617) 247-8611/E-mail: radhagopi@juno.com

Chicago, Illinois — 1716 W. Lunt Ave., 60626/ Tel. (773) 973-0900/ Fax: (773) 973-0526/ E-mail: chicago@iskcon.net

Columbus, Ohio — 379 W. Eighth Ave., 43201/ Tel. (614) 421-1661/ Fax: (614) 294-0545/ E-mail: malati.acbsp@pamho.net

♦ **Dallas, Texas** — 5430 Gurley Ave., 75223/ Tel. (214) 827-6330/ Fax: (214) 823-7264/ E-mail: txkrishnas@aol.com; restaurant: vegetariantaste@aol.com

♦ **Denver, Colorado** — 1400 Cherry St., 80220/ Tel. (303) 333-5461/ Fax: (303) 321-9052/ E-mail: naikatma.acbsp@pamho.net

♦ **Detroit, Michigan** — 383 Lenox Ave., 48215/ Tel. (313) 824-6000/ Fax: (313) 822-3748/ E-mail: girigovardhana@hotmail.com

Gainesville, Florida — 214 N.W. 14th St., 32603/ Tel. (352) 336-4183/ Fax: (352) 379-2923/ E-mail: krishna@afn.org

Hartford, Connecticut — 1683 Main St., E. Hartford 06108/ Tel. & fax: (860) 289-7252/ E-mail: pyarimohan@aol.com

♦ **Honolulu, Hawaii** — 51 Coelho Way, 96817/ Tel. (808) 595-3947/ E-mail: vrnda@aol.com

Houston, Texas — 1320 W. 34th St., 77018/ Tel. (713) 686-4482/ Fax: (713) 956-9968/ E-mail: mbalar@ev1.net

Kansas City, Missouri — Rupanuga Vedic College (Men's Seminary), 5201 The Paseo, 64110/ Tel. (800) 340-5286/ Fax: (816) 361-0509/ E-mail: info@rvc.edu

♦ **Laguna Beach, California** — 285 Legion St., 92651/ Tel. (949) 494-7029/ E-mail: tuka108@hotmail.com

Las Vegas, Nevada — 5226 Sandstone Dr., 89142/ Tel. (702) 440-4998/ E-mail: surapala@pamho.net

Long Island, New York — 197 S. Ocean Avenue, Freeport 11520/ Tel. (516) 223-4909/ E-mail: garuda@optonline.net

♦ **Los Angeles, California** — 3764 Watseka Ave., 90034/ Tel. (310) 836-2676/ Fax: (310) 839-2715/ E-mail: nirantara@juno.com

Los Angeles, California — 3520–3526 Slauson Ave., 90043/ Tel. (323) 295-1517/ E-mail: Mr.Wisdomla@aol.com

♦ **Miami, Florida** — 3220 Virginia St., 33133 (mail: P.O. Box 337, Coconut Grove, FL 33233)/ Tel. (305) 442-7218/ Fax: (305) 444-7145

New Orleans, Louisiana — 2936 Esplanade Ave., 70119/ Tel. (504) 486-3583/ E-mail: rrk196820@cs.com

♦ **New York, New York** — 305 Schermerhorn St., Brooklyn 11217/ Tel. (718) 855-6714/ Fax: (718) 875-6127/ E-mail: ramabhadra@aol.com

New York, New York — 26 Second Avenue, 10003/ Tel. (212) 420-1130/ E-mail: dayananda@msn.com

Philadelphia, Pennsylvania — 41 West Allens Lane, 19119/ Tel. (215) 247-4600/ Fax: (215) 247-8702/ E-mail: iskconphilly@aol.com

Philadelphia, Pennsylvania — 1408 South St., 19146/ Tel. (215) 985-9335/ E-mail: savecows@aol.com

Phoenix, Arizona — 100 S. Weber Dr., Chandler 85226/ Tel. (480) 705-4900/ Fax: (480) 705-4901/ E-mail: svgd108@yahoo.com

Portland, Oregon — 3766 SE Divsion, 97202/ Tel. (503) 236-6734/ E-mail: iskconoregon@hotmail.com

Queens, New York — 114-37 Lefferts Blvd., 11420 / Tel. & fax: (718) 848-9010 / E-mail: sunandanadas@hotmail.com

♦ **St. Louis, Missouri** — 3926 Lindell Blvd., 63108/ Tel. (314) 535-8085/ Fax: (314) 535-0672/ E-mail: temple@harekrishna-stl.com

♦ **San Diego, California** — 1030 Grand Ave., Pacific Beach 92109/ Tel. (858) 483-2500/ Fax: (858) 483-0941/ E-mail: gandharvika@pamho.net

San Jose, California — 2990 Union Ave., 95124/ Tel. (408) 559-3197/ Fax: (408) 369-8073/ E-mail: bhvatsala@hotmail.com

Seattle, Washington — 1420 228th Ave. S.E., Sammamish 98075/ Tel. (425) 391-3293/ Fax: (425) 868-8928/ E-mail: iskconseattle@yahoo.com

♦ Temples with restaurants or dining

Tallahassee, Florida — 1323 Nylic St., 32304/ Tel. & fax: (850) 224-3803/ E-mail: darudb@hotmail.com
Tampa, Florida — 14610 North 17th St., Lutz 33549/ Tel. (813) 971-6474/ E-mail: krishnaram108@hotmail.com
Towaco, New Jersey — 100 Jacksonville Rd. (mail: P.O. Box 109), 07082/ Tel. & fax: (973) 299-0970/ E-mail: newjersey@iskcon.net
♦ **Tucson, Arizona** — 711 E. Blacklidge Dr., 85719/ Tel. (520) 792-0630/ Fax: (520) 791-0906/ E-mail: tucphx@cs.com
Washington, D.C. — 10310 Oaklyn Dr., Potomac, Maryland 20854/ Tel. (301) 299-2100/ Fax: (301) 299-5025/ E-mail: sri.trikalajna.mg@pamho.net

RURAL COMMUNITIES

Carriere, Mississippi (New Talavan) — 31492 Anner Road, 39426/ Tel. (601) 749-9460 or 799-1354/ Fax: (601) 799-2924/ Fax: (601) 799-2924/ E-mail: talavan@mypicayune.com
Gurabo, Puerto Rico (New Govardhana Hill) — Carr. 181, Km. 16.3, Bo. Santa Rita, Gurabo
(mail: HC-01, Box 8440, Gurabo, PR 00778)/ (Office) Tel. & fax: (787) 737-4265/ (Temple) Tel. (787)712-0358/ E-mail: iskconpr@hotmail.com
Hillsborough, North Carolina (New Goloka) — 1032 Dimmocks Mill Rd., 27278/ Tel. (919) 732-6492/ Fax: (919) 732-8033/ E-mail: bkgoswami@compuserve.com
♦ **Moundsville, West Virginia (New Vrindaban)** — R.D. No. 1, Box 319, Hare Krishna Ridge, 26041/ Tel. (304) 843-1600; Guest House, (304) 845-5905/ Fax: (304) 854-0023/ E-mail: newvrindaban@yahoo.com
Mulberry, Tennessee (Murari-sevaka) — Rt. No. 1, Box 146-A, 37359/ Tel. (931) 759-4884/ Fax: (615) 759-5785/ E-mail: visnujana@hotmail.com
Port Royal, Pennsylvania (Gita Nagari) — R.D. No. 1, Box 839, 17082/ Tel. & fax: (717) 527-4101/ E-mail: vrajalila@acsworld.net
Sandy Ridge, North Carolina — 1264 Prabhupada Rd., 27046/ Tel. (336) 593-9888

ADDITIONAL RESTAURANTS

Gainesville, Florida — Radha's Vegetarian Cafe, 125 NW 23rd Ave., Suite 17, 32609/ Tel. (352) 378-2955
San Juan, Puerto Rico — Gopal, 201B Calle Tetuan, Viejo San Juan, 00901/ Tel. (787) 724-0229
Seattle, Washington — My Sweet Lord, 5521 University Way, 98105/ Tel. (425) 643-4664
Tallahassee, Florida — Higher Taste, 411 St. Francis St., 32301/ Tel. (850) 894-4296

AUSTRALASIA

AUSTRALIA

Adelaide — 25 Le Hunte St., Kilburn, SA 5084/ Tel. +61 (08) 8359-5120/ Fax: (08) 8359-5149
Brisbane — 95 Bank Rd., Graceville (mail: P.O. Box 83, Indurupilly), QLD 4068/ Tel. +61 (07) 3379-5455/ Fax: +61 (07) 3379-5880
Canberra — 1 Quick St., Ainslie, ACT 2602 (mail: P.O. Box 1411, Canberra, ACT 2601)/ Tel. & fax: +61 (02) 6262-6208/ E-mail: adi@actweb.net
Melbourne — 197 Danks St. (mail: P.O. Box 125), Albert Park , VIC 3206/ Tel. +61 (03) 9699-5122/ Fax: +61 (03) 9690-4093/ E-mail: iskcon@bigpond.net.au
Newcastle — 28 Bull St., Mayfield, NSW 2304/ Tel. +61 (02) 4967-7000/ E-mail: iskcon_newcastle@yahoo.com.au
Perth — 144 Railway Parade (corner of The Strand) [mail: P.O. Box 102], Bayswater, WA 6053/ Tel. +61 (08) 9370-1552/ Fax: +61 (08) 9272-6636/ E-mail: perth@pamho.net
Sydney — 180 Falcon St., North Sydney, NSW 2060 (mail: P.O. Box 459, Cammeray, NSW 2062)/ Tel. +61 (029) 9959-4558/ Fax: +61 (029) 9957-1893

RURAL COMMUNITIES

Bambra (New Nandagram) — 50 Seaches Outlet, off 1265 Winchelsea Deans Marsh Rd., Bambra VIC 3241/ Tel. +61 (03) 5288-7383/ E-mail: iskcon@bigpond.net.au
Cessnock, NSW — New Gokula Farm, Lewis Lane (off Mount View Rd., Millfield, near Cessnock [mail: P.O. Box 399, Cessnock]), NSW
2325/ Tel. +61 (02) 4998-800/ Fax: (Sydney temple)
Murwillumbah (New Govardhana) — Tyalgum Rd., Eungella (mail: P.O. Box 685), NSW 2484/ Tel. & fax: +61 (02) 6672-6579/ Fax: +61 (02) 6672-5498

RESTAURANTS

Adelaide — Hare Krishna Food for Life, 79 Hindley St., SA 5000/ Tel. +61 (08) 8231-5258
Brisbane — Govinda's, 99 Elizabeth St., 1st floor, QLD 4000/ Tel. +61 (07) 3210-0255
Brisbane — Hare Krishna Food for Life, 190 Brunswick St., Fortitude Valley, QLD/ Tel. +61 (07) 3854-1016/ E-mail: brisbane@pamho.net
Melbourne — Crossways, 1st Floor, 123 Swanston St., VIC 3000/ Tel. +61 (03) 9650-2939
Melbourne — Gopal's, 139 Swanston St., VIC 3000/ Tel. +61 (03) 9650-1578
New Castle — Krishna's Vegetarian Cafe, 110 King Street, corner of King & Wolf Streets, NSW 2300/ Tel. +61 (02) 4929-6900
Perth — Hare Krishna Food for Life, 200 William St., Northbridge, WA 6003/ Tel. +61 (08) 9227-1684/ E-mail: perth@pamho.net
Sydney — Govinda's Upstairs,112 Darlinghurst Road, Darlinghurst NSW 2010/ Tel. +61 (02) 9380-5155
Sydney — Hare Krishna Food for Life, 529B King St., Newtown, NSW 2042/ Tel. +61 (02) 9550-6524

NEW ZEALAND

Christchurch, NZ — 83 Bealey Ave. (mail: P.O. Box 25-190)/ Tel. +64 (03) 366-5174/
Fax: +64 (03) 366-1965/ E-mail: iskconchch@clear.net.nz
Wellington, NZ — 105 Newlands Rd., Newlands (mail: P.O. Box 2753)/ Tel. +64 (04) 478-1414

RURAL COMMUNITY

Auckland, NZ (New Varshan) — Hwy. 28, Riverhead, next to Huapai Golf Course (mail: R.D. 2, Kumeu)/ Tel. +64 (09) 412-8075/ Fax: +64 (09) 412-7130

RESTAURANTS

Auckland, NZ — Hare Krishna Food for Life, 268 Karangahape Road/ Tel. +64 (09) 300-7585

Stay in touch with Krishna

Read more from *Back to Godhead* magazine—
6 months for only $9.95! (Offer valid in US only.)

SPECIAL TRIAL OFFER!

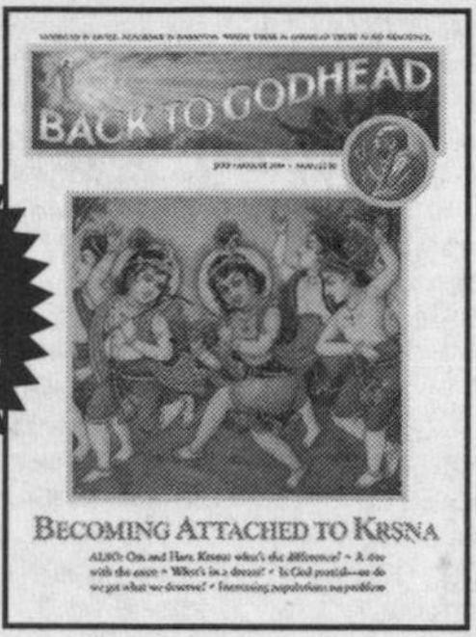

YES, please send me *Back to Godhead* magazine.

❒ Enter my subscription for 6 months (3 issues) for only $9.95 (US only, please)

❒ Enter my subscription for 1 year (6 issues) for only $17.95 (save 25% off the cover price). For Canada, add $3. All other countries, add $9. (Payment must be in US funds drawn on a US bank.)

❒ Bill me ❒ Payment enclosed ❒ Credit card

Name ______________________________

Address ______________________ Tel. ________

City ______________ ST ________ Zip ________

Card no. ______________________ Exp. date _____

Signature ______________________________

Mail or fax this coupon to:

BTG Service Center, P.O. Box 430, Alachua, FL 32616-0430, USA

For faster service, call toll free: 1-800-800-3284